HOLDING

on to

NORMAL

*How I Survived Cancer
and Made It to the Other Side,
Happier, Healthier and Stronger*

ALANA SOMERVILLE

PUBLISHED BY SIMON & SCHUSTER

New York   London   Toronto   Sydney   New Delhi

Simon & Schuster Canada
A Division of Simon & Schuster, Inc.
166 King Street East, Suite 300
Toronto, Ontario M5A 1J3

This Simon & Schuster Canada edition May 2018

For information about special discounts for bulk purchases,
please contact Simon & Schuster Special Sales at 1-800-268-3216
or CustomerService@simonandschuster.ca.

Library and Archives Canada Cataloguing in Publication

Somerville, Alana
[Chemosabe]
Holding on to normal : how I survived cancer and made it to the other
side, happier, healthier and stronger / Alana Somerville.

Originally published under title: Chemosabe : cancer warrior.
Issued in print and electronic formats.
ISBN 978-1-5011-6812-3 (hardcover).—ISBN 978-1-5011-6814-7 (ebook)

1. Somerville, Alana—Health. 2. Breast—Cancer—Patients—Biography.
I. Title. II. Title: Chemosabe.

RC280.B8S64 2018 362.19699'4490092 C2017-906516-5
C2017-906517-3

Manufactured in the United States of America

1 3 5 7 9 10 8 6 4 2

ISBN 978-1-5011-6812-3
ISBN 978-1-5011-6814-7 (ebook)

All photographs in the insert are courtesy of the author, except as marked.

This is for my children, Charley and Rudy.
I fight for you, in the hopes that you will never
have to wage this war.

This is also for Talia.
You were the strongest warrior I've ever known.
I continue this fight for you.

Contents

$\mathcal{S}$

Foreword

ℒ

I met Alana in Toronto during Breast Cancer Awareness Month, October 2014. She gave me a copy of this book, *Holding on to Normal,* and I started it that evening on my flight to New York. I read without pause to the end. I felt drained but enlightened as I journeyed with Alana in her fight against this terrible disease.

While it's not pure enjoyment, it's a captivating and riveting read that inspires and instills hope. I urge everyone to read it, in order to truly know what it means to be diagnosed with breast cancer.

We all hope we never go through it, although one woman in eight will. Alana's book has inspired me to continue raising funds and awareness for breast cancer, and I commend her bravery in sharing her experience with us.

ELIZABETH HURLEY

PROLOGUE

Everything changed the summer of 2010.

We had just returned from a week at our friend's cottage up north near Haliburton, Ontario—my husband, Greg; our three-and-a-half-year-old daughter, Charley; our six-month-old son, Rudy; and me. We normally would go up north at least once or twice a summer. We would fish, jump off the dock, swim in the river and have bonfires at night.

The time away had been wonderful, as usual, especially because it allowed me to step away from my life at home, which always seemed so busy. I'm the type of person who can't sit still. Whenever I do, a little voice in my head runs through all the things I could be or should be doing. I've always found it impossible to leave things until another day. Going up north forced me to do just that. Even the kids had extra eyes on them, so I could relax and breathe in a way I could never do at home. And I'd also begun weaning Rudy, cutting out a couple of feedings during the day and replacing them with formula. The new routine seemed to be working well for both of us.

Basically, my life was perfect. I had everything I had ever wanted. I was married, with two beautiful children. My husband and I had built a house with a pool in a quiet little neighborhood with great neighbors. I was the only one out of three children in my family whose first house was a brand-new one. I had a job as a teacher, loved my work colleagues and had good ties with friends. I was healthy, Greg was healthy, my kids were healthy.

Two years before our cottage trip, though, I began questioning things. Could my life really be going so well? What if there was a threat I couldn't see? While it sounds weird in retrospect, I think I had a gut feeling that someday something would go wrong. In 2008, when I was thirty-one years old, I decided I needed to have a mammogram.

Of course my doctor questioned my reasoning. "Why do you want to do that? Do you have a family history?" he asked.

That was reasonable. In fact, I had no family history of breast cancer other than a maternal great-aunt who'd had it. And my doctor didn't actually consider that to constitute a family history.

"I realize I'm way too young to get breast cancer, and I'm very low risk," I said. I also knew that breastfeeding my daughter for nine months reduced my breast cancer risk. And I ate healthily, I exercised, and I didn't smoke.

So why did I want to have a mammogram?

"I've heard that having a baseline record of breast health could be useful if anything ever comes up in the future," I said.

My doctor nodded, not entirely convinced, but at least listening. In the end, he sent me to a breast screening clinic at the local hospital for a mammogram. "Just so you know," he warned, "it might hurt a bit. You okay with that?"

"Sure," I said. "No problem."

He was right. It did hurt a bit. But it wasn't so bad, at least for me. The end result? My breasts were a little dense, which is common in young women. Most important, though, they were normal. Wonderful! That was exactly what I wanted to hear, and I felt reassured. Life truly was great.

And life remained great two years later. After we returned home from the cottage, the whole family settled into our usual routine. As I continued to wean Rudy, my breasts produced less milk. Rudy still woke for his regular four A.M. feeding, and the night everything changed—Saturday, August 21, 2010—was no exception. As I picked Rudy up and placed him on the pillow on my lap, I eased into the routine of feeding. I always felt lucky to have the bonding experience of breastfeeding, something that fathers miss out on—although I would have preferred to bond at a more reasonable hour of the day.

I cuddled Rudy's body close to mine, soaking in that special baby smell as he nursed. I looked down at his satisfied little face, and I couldn't help but smile. He looked just like my daughter, Charley, had as a baby and yet was himself. I shifted him and that's when my world stopped.

I felt a lump in my breast.

Part One

SHOCK

Chapter 1

BEFORE AND AFTER

∽

I *divide my life* into two parts: before I was diagnosed with breast cancer and after.

Before, I worried that other people around me would have to go through heartbreak, illness or grief, and that I'd have to find the courage to help them. I also thought I'd live to be older than a lot of my family members, and I worried about ending up alone, because surely I was the heartiest, the strongest. Surely I'd be the last to go. In hindsight, this seems a little shortsighted, because it never occurred to me I could be faced with anything difficult. It would only be *someone else*. Nothing bad would happen to *me*.

Now I was fully awake. I put Rudy back in his crib and examined myself more thoroughly. Was my other breast like this? No, it wasn't. When did this lump show up? How long had it been there without my noticing? What was I supposed to do now, in the middle of the night? How could I tell my husband about it without making him nervous?

An even better question was, How would I tell my mother? She had just had a biopsy herself six months before, but fortunately, the results had come back clear. It had been a tough time for all of us as we waited for those results. The thought of losing my mom had rocked me to the core. Now I couldn't help but think to myself, *Here we go again.*

I imagined what I would say to her. "Hey, Mom, I know it sounds silly, but I have this tiny lump in my breast, so I thought I should get it checked out. Probably nothing. Probably due to breastfeeding." That's what I'd say. I would downplay it for her, because this was nothing we needed to be worried about.

I thought about my friends, too. I wanted to ask them if they'd ever had lumps like this. After all, most of them had breastfed within the last couple of years or were doing it now. This *must* have happened to them, too. They just didn't tell me about it.

I tried to breathe, to not imagine the worst. But it was so hard. How could I possibly fall back asleep again? I thought about those whispers, that gut feeling I'd had two years before. But the mammogram was clear, I told myself. I clung to those results. They couldn't be wrong. Nothing could be wrong.

I paced up and down the hallway. It was the weekend—how could I possibly wait till Monday to call my doctor? The first family doctor I had consulted, Doctor 1, the one who had hesitated about sending me for a mammogram but eventually did, had subsequently been replaced by a new doctor, Doctor 2. (Little did I know it at the time, but there would soon be many more doctors in my life.) I had much more confidence in this doctor, but after all, it was Sunday morning. It wasn't like I could call for reassurance. But I'd had a full physical by Doctor 2 just two months earlier, and he had given me a clean bill of health. He didn't examine my breasts, though, because I was breastfeeding—or at least that's what I assumed. I did remember what he said at the end of the checkup: "You have a passport to old age."

After much more pacing, I crawled back into bed beside Greg. I was shivering. I tried to sneak in close to him to warm up, but the shaking wouldn't stop. I wasn't cold. I was in shock. I felt so alone. I couldn't clear my mind. I thought about every worst-case scenario. I tried to reason with myself, but it was impossible.

It was one of the longest nights of my life.

> I thought about every worst-case scenario. I tried to reason with myself, but it was impossible. It was one of the longest nights of my life.

༄

When I woke up and came out of our bedroom the next morning, Greg was in the kitchen. I joined him and poured myself a coffee, trying to think of what to say to him. My hand trembled as I poured some milk into my steaming cup. When I told Greg, I couldn't look at him. In some small way—I can't explain why—I felt embarrassed.

"I found a lump," I said. I didn't feel the need to explain.

"When?"

"Last night when I got up to feed Rudy." Still, I couldn't look at him.

"Can you show me?" he asked, concern in his voice.

I took off my bra and guided Greg's hand to the spot, hoping he wouldn't feel it, hoping it had disappeared.

But it hadn't.

"I'm sure it's nothing," he said. "Try not to worry. It probably has something to do with the fact that you're starting to wean Rudy. But go get it checked out."

Greg was always interested in medical situations because he was a volunteer firefighter—he usually had lots to say. The fact that he didn't this time kind of worried me. I was looking for reassurance.

I called my mother and gave her my planned lines. She was worried right away. "When did you find it?" she asked, and the questions continued from there. "When did you check your breasts last time? Is it hard? Where is it exactly? Does it hurt? Can you breastfeed?"

I answered as best I could. "I don't remember the last time I checked my breasts. I'm breastfeeding, but less now. No one told me to check them while I'm breastfeeding. They're huge and uncomfortable, and the last thing I want to do is feel them. It's on my lower left side. It doesn't hurt. Rudy has been losing interest lately. Do you think that's why?" I was starting to panic, but she reminded me that I'd had mastitis in my early breastfeeding days with Charley and suggested it could be that.

This was different, though. Mastitis was painful; this lump wasn't. When I had mastitis, my breasts had been warm and red, as if there was an infection, and that wasn't the case now, either.

"You should call your doctor right away tomorrow morning."

"Of course," I said. I hung up. I fed the kids, then went into the living room with them.

"Mommy, you're not paying attention!" Charley sounded just like me when I scolded her, but she was right: I simply couldn't focus on the game she wanted to play. I turned on the television, found one of Charley's favorite shows, then snuggled up with her on the couch, hoping she wouldn't notice how distracted I was. We snuggled for about twenty minutes, but that's as long as it lasted.

"Let's go for a swim," Charley said.

I didn't feel like it, but I knew it would make the time pass.

"All right, go get your bathing suit. I'll get Rudy ready." Rudy wasn't walking yet, so I had to get him set up in the bouncy chair outside. I knew we wouldn't be out for long—Rudy would start crying, and Charley couldn't be left alone in the water. But Greg joined us outside a short while later and kept Charley happy in the pool while I fed Rudy. We spent most of the day playing out there, but I couldn't stop thinking about that lump.

That night I had dinner with friends and told them.

"I remember a similar situation when I was breastfeeding," one of them said. "My doctor gave me antibiotics and told me to ice the lump and come back in two weeks. It disappeared. Yours will, too. Don't worry."

I hoped so.

That evening after I got home from dinner, I was edgy. I was anxious. I was downright irritable. It was impossible to sleep, and even though I tried not to think about the lump in my breast, it was futile.

Monday morning finally came, and I phoned the office of Doctor 2 as soon as it opened.

"Good morning. May I help you?" the nurse on the line answered.

"Hi, it's Alana Somerville. I need to make an appointment with the doctor." My voice was calm and polite, but I wasn't feeling calm at all. I wanted to just show up at the office right away. I wanted to get in to see him right that second. I didn't care if anyone else had a sore throat or an ingrown toenail. This was me, and it was important. But I knew yelling through the phone and demanding I be a top priority wouldn't help get me in sooner. One of the most important life lessons my mother taught me was to ask for what you want in the nicest way possible until you get it.

"He doesn't have anything available until Friday. Does that work?"

"It doesn't," I said, remaining calm. "I've just discovered a lump in my breast. I'm very concerned and I'm going to come in today to be looked at. What time can I come in?"

There was a pause at the other end of the line. "How about three o'clock?"

That was exactly the response I was hoping for. My jaw unclenched. I could actually breathe for a moment. I had an appointment.

Chapter 2

FALLING APART

ℐ

Waiting for my appointment felt like an eternity. Once I got to the office, I waited forty-five minutes to be called in, and another fifteen minutes in the exam room. I was impatient, to say the least, and the minutes felt like hours. I tried flipping through fashion magazines to distract myself, but my hands were too shaky and I wasn't even interested in looking at photos or reading the articles. The bra advertisements also kept reminding me of the reason I was there, so I closed the magazine and slapped it down on the table, frustrated. Finally, in came Doctor 2. A nurse practitioner followed him in. I figured she was probably there because the doctor would be examining my breast. I had never had my breasts examined before—the only time someone in the medical field had touched my breasts was during that first mammogram, two years prior.

⸜

"I understand you noticed a lump?" Doctor 2 said.

"Yes, and I know it wasn't there before."

He carefully examined my breast. I stared at a medical poster on the wall as his fingers pushed into my flesh. I stared at the tongue compressors and cotton balls in the jars on the counter. He was kneading now, searching. I looked at at the ceiling tiles, noticing where the leaks were and how the ceiling tile in the corner didn't quite fit properly. For some reason, I didn't want to make eye contact with him, possibly because I was scared I'd see a reaction on his face. I also felt embarrassed—I was being touched in an intimate place by a virtual stranger. Why was this happening to me?

"Here," he said at last. "This is the spot." I think he was speaking to me, but at the same time it seemed like he was having a dialogue with himself, talking himself through the examination. He indicated an area in the lower left quadrant of my left breast. He had found the lump—which meant it was indeed there and was big enough for him to feel. I felt as though my life rested in his hands. I looked at him for the first time.

"I'm glad it's movable," he said. "That means it's not attached to your breastbone."

What if it was? What would that mean? I was too shaken to ask those questions out loud.

"I'm going to refer you for an ultrasound and a mammogram to rule out anything sinister," he said.

I knew in the back of my head that this "sinister" thing he was talking about was the dreaded C-word, but I couldn't quite absorb that. The exam was over, and I was told I could get dressed, so I did. I left the office without asking any questions at all. *This can't possibly be happening to me,* I thought as I walked down the street towards my car.

⸜

The days that followed between my consultation with Doctor 2 and the mammogram and ultrasound were brutal. I was in a daze and kept telling myself this must be a mistake. I sat at my computer, researching all the possible scenarios that could play out, but that was the wrong thing to do. I got redirected to website after website about cancer. Everything pointed to cancer.

My mother came over to visit on the next Saturday.

"Everything okay, Alana?" She was helping me tidy up in the kitchen, and I'd dropped a dish while I was putting things in the dishwasher.

"Fine, Mom. My hands are just wet." But they weren't. I was trying to behave as though everything was normal while I was falling apart on the inside. In a sort of vicious circle, everyone around me was trying to stay positive, too.

And in the midst of everything, I was trying to come to grips with potty training Charley. "Charley, you're all wet!" I yelled one time when I realized that she'd had yet another accident. I was holding Rudy, who was screaming, and I was absolutely beside myself. Mom had just dropped by for another visit. She took Rudy from me.

"You need to relax, Alana." Her voice was kind and quiet as she said it, but I almost started crying. Everyone was worked up, but I knew *I* was the cause. I was more affected than I'd realized—and the worst was yet to come.

♪

The following Tuesday finally arrived, and with it my appointments. The mammogram was first. As a school teacher, I meet and get to know many people, and the technician happened to be the parent of one of my past students. I seemed to run into her all the time at the hospital—she had also performed my previous mammogram.

"How are you?" I asked.

"Great! How are the kids?"

"Oh, you know. Charley's potty training, and I don't know if I'm going to survive." I thought about the couple of days a week that Charley went to day care. It was all that was saving me right now.

The tech laughed, then explained the procedure and got me into position. As I stood there, attempting to breathe but not move, my breast mashed between the mammogram plates, I tried hard to get information out of her. Could she see anything? I knew she was a technician, not a doctor, and wasn't supposed to tell me my results, but that didn't matter. I was hoping that if she noticed something right away, she would tell me, since we knew each other. She wasn't talking, though. I waited patiently while she looked at the films to make sure they'd turned out, and then she finally spoke.

"I don't see anything." Big sigh of relief. She couldn't see any tumors, which meant that maybe there weren't any. That was good, right? I gathered my things, and she walked me to my next appointment and introduced me to the ultrasound technician. Before she left, though, she stopped to talk with the tech. I strained to hear what they were saying but couldn't. *Was* there something in my breast that wasn't supposed to be there?

The ultrasound tech gave me a gown and left while I got changed, then came back in. "If you could just lie back on the table," she said. She had me expose my breast.

"This is going to be cold." She squirted gel on me and used a wand-like instrument to rub it around while she stared past me at a black-and-white screen. I craned my neck and tried to see what I could and, again, asked every question I could possibly think of: "What is that black shadow there? Is that the lump? What are you looking at now?"

The technician was surprisingly chatty, but not in an upbeat way, more in an investigative way. I remembered with my pregnancy ultrasounds that the technicians were usually deep in thought. She asked me a bunch of questions: When did you find the lump? Does it hurt? Has it grown since you found it? Maybe if she hadn't spoken at all, I wouldn't have been so alarmed. It wasn't that she said anything in particular, but I could feel something was definitely wrong.

After she had finished and handed me a large wad of tissue to wipe the gel off with, she told me I'd have to wait about a week for both the results of the mammogram and the ultrasound. I couldn't believe it. A week? That amount of time sounded like torture to me! I left the appointment feeling overwhelmed, confused and angry.

On Friday, just three days after my mammogram and ultrasound, Rudy was in his high chair and I was feeding him when the phone rang. Call display is a great thing. I could see that it was the doctor's office. I snatched up the receiver.

"Hi, is Alana Somerville there, please?"

It was Doctor 2. *Oh, shit. It can't be good if the doctor is calling himself.*

"The results of the tests were somewhat concerning," he began.

I put Rudy's spoon down.

"I suggest you meet with a surgeon and get a biopsy done, again just to rule out anything sinister."

"Okay," I said, and we ended the conversation with the doctor explaining that the surgeon's office would call me with an appointment.

As I hung up, it hit me. I slumped in front of Rudy in his high chair, and all my courage faded away. Tears came in full force. I was overwhelmed with fear. Sweet little Rudy just stared at me. What was he thinking? He couldn't possibly have any idea what was going on. I sobbed and sobbed, angry thoughts seething in my head. *This should not be happening to me. I have the two most beautiful children and this can't be happening to me. My children need me. I don't have time to be sick!*

Greg continued to tell me things would be fine. "It's probably nothing," he said.

I looked at him, wanting to sink into his arms, wanting desperately to believe what he was saying. "I hope you're right."

He hugged me. "I'm sure it's nothing, Alana."

"I know you're trying to make me feel better, but I can't help but worry," I said. I wasn't just worried, though—I was terrified. How could he possibly know what was going on?

Everyone I talked to—Greg; my brother, Braden; my sister, Erin; my friends—seemed to dismiss the fact that there could be a problem, and those dismissals irritated me. I couldn't help but think that it's a lot easier to say things will be fine when you aren't the one going for a biopsy.

My mother was the exception. After all, she had just had a biopsy not that long before. She was the only person who seemed to be taking what was happening seriously, who didn't just dismiss it. Her advice was simple: "You'll cross each bridge as you come to it. If you worry now and it turns out to be nothing, you've worried for nothing. If it turns out to be something and you're worried now, you'll have worried twice." It must have been difficult for her, but she was there for me every step of the way—even if she was treading carefully around me like everyone else. Her voice had the appropriate amount of fear, too, even though she seemed to be the one who was trying to hide it the most.

When I called certain friends or family members, they avoided the topic, saying things like "Quite the weather we've been having, no?" or "Hey, did I tell you about the family trip we're going on next month?" Some people told me about cancer patients they'd known who went on to live long and happy lives. One of my friends told me a story about a young boy who'd been diagnosed with cancer and was on his deathbed. "I don't think he's going to make it," she confessed in hushed tones. I tried to change the subject, but deep down, I felt the impact. If this could happen to a young boy, could it happen to me? Then I got mad. How *dare* she compare me to someone who was dying? I wasn't going to die!

All of the responses to my news begged the question: How did I want people to respond? What is the "right" way to respond to the news that someone has a lump that may or may not be cancerous? I honestly didn't know, and to this day, I still don't. I had no clue what I wanted to hear from anyone. Nothing anyone could say was going to change what was happening to me. I didn't want easy denials—a pat on the head and a superficial "everything will be fine." Maybe that was the way most people coped—by pretending that the worst wasn't possible. And maybe the people who didn't say anything to me at all didn't know what to say; that happened to be their way of coping. I just knew that few people were saying anything that helped.

Dealing with this was bringing me down. I had to put on a brave face. If anyone had asked me—truly asked—how I felt, I would have said: I feel disheartened. I feel alone. I feel hopeless. Help!

Chapter 3

STUPID PINK EVERYWHERE

Maybe because the next month was October, which happens to be Breast Cancer Awareness month, all of a sudden, everywhere I looked I saw pink. Everything I saw and heard pointed to the fact that breast cancer was in my world. Every commercial on the television seemed to be about raising money for breast cancer. I ordered a new pair of running shoes, and the only color they came in was white with a pink stripe. Every product I looked at seemed to have that damn pink ribbon on it. Everything screamed breast cancer at me.

It felt surreal. I was filled with anxiety, and not one minute of the day went by when I wasn't thinking about my fate, even though only just over two weeks had passed since I'd first found the lump. Yet I had to keep myself together because I had kids to take care of, a house to run, and medical appointments to get myself to. It felt like I was living two different lives, but simultaneously.

Things were moving fairly quickly, though. I was already up to Doctor 3. I wanted to keep track—so it felt simpler to just refer to them as numbers to keep everything straight.

Doctor 3 was a local surgeon. We met for a consultation before the biopsy was performed. Yet again I had to disrobe from the waist up, and yet again I waited alone in an exam room, cold, semi-naked, with only a hospital gown as protection between me and the help I needed. Doctor 3 examined me, focusing in on the lump.

"Is this concerning to you?" I asked.

"Yes, it is," he answered. Could he have been more blunt? Could he not have beaten around the bush a little and given me some hope?

"We need to do a biopsy to see exactly what it is we are dealing with here. I'll try to get you in within the next week."

I didn't ask much after that. I got dressed and slowly walked out to the reception area, where a nurse took my information and said she would get back to me with a biopsy date. She called later that day. The biopsy would be done by Doctor 4 in the hospital. It was scheduled for Friday, September 10, three weeks after I'd found the lump. Doctor 3 would meet with me again after the biopsy to discuss the results.

I felt shell-shocked. I thought about who would come with me to the biopsy appointment. I didn't want to go alone. My mother, I decided. She was tough, probably the toughest woman I knew, even though she had a habit of crying while watching sappy commercials. I wanted her there with me, but she was also the best person to watch the children. In the end, Greg came with me, while Mom watched the kids.

We walked into the hospital, and I was already feeling as though the antiseptic smell and white walls were becoming a recurrent theme in my life. I hoped I wouldn't run into anyone I knew. I had that embarrassed feeling again. I couldn't quite wrap my head around it. Why would *I* be embarrassed? What did I have to hide? And yet all I wanted to do was hide. I wasn't ready to discuss with acquaintances what was going on in my life.

Close family and friends, yes; acquaintances, no. Illogical as it sounds, I felt like I had done something wrong to end up in this predicament. And I didn't want people to start talking about me.

> I had that embarrassed feeling again. I couldn't quite wrap my head around it. Why would *I* be embarrassed? What did I have to hide? And yet all I wanted to do was hide.

When the nurse called my name, it was clear I would have to leave Greg in the waiting room. How I wished he could come with me. I changed—stripping was by then becoming routine—and waited till the nurse came to lead me into the operating room. Another table, more exposure. I felt cold, but that could have just been my fear. On the wall, an anatomy chart of a dissected woman stared me down. I could relate to her—exposed and vulnerable, her privacy and dignity cut away. I tried to cover myself with the thin sheet of blue paper I'd been given, but it felt wholly inadequate. I felt as though my privacy and dignity had been sliced away.

Doctor 4, the radiologist who would perform the biopsy, entered along with a nurse, and they got right to business. My breast was frozen with a few jabs of a needle full of local anesthetic. Then an ultrasound was used to find the exact location of the lump. The doctor took a device that when it was employed sounded disconcertingly like a staple gun and used it to remove three samples of tissue from the lump.

The process didn't hurt at all, which surprised me. I thought that if someone had been jabbing my breast with a machine sounding like a staple gun, I would definitely feel a throbbing pain. Instead, there was just a little pressure. I found the sound of the machine more alarming than anything else. Doctor 4 showed the bits of tissue to me when it was all over. They were in a container filled with liquid and were each about the width of a small juice box straw. The sight of pieces of my breast floating in front of me made me a tiny bit woozy. Could so much be learned from samples so small?

"Here's an ice pack," the nurse said. "It's to put in your bra when you get dressed. And take Tylenol for the pain."

I sat up. I wasn't concerned about the pain. "How long will it take to get the results?"

"Between seven and ten days."

Again I would have to wait. I found waiting the most awful part of everything. Waiting was when my mind wandered, when I thought about all of the negatives and the possibilities. If the results were negative, were they really negative? Or would they tell me later that they'd made a mistake? If they were positive, what next?

The following Tuesday, four days later, I received a call from the surgeon's office saying that the results were in. No one would tell me anything over the phone; the receptionist simply scheduled an appointment with the doctor for the next day at nine A.M. Surely, if the biopsy results weren't troubling, the appointment could have waited for the following week? I thought about all that pink I kept seeing, about cancer, and felt overcome by dread.

Wednesday, September 15. I circled the day on my calendar. Would it be the day that would change my life forever?

Chapter 4

DIAGNOSIS

S*ometimes more than* one person is needed on a journey. Both my husband and mother accompanied me to get the results of the biopsy.

We didn't have to wait long before Doctor 3 came into the office, sat down and began to tell me my fate. I don't think he even said hello. His words came as if in slow motion, yet somehow so fast.

"It looks like it's cancer," he said.

I couldn't move. I replayed his words in my head. Cancer. I had known all along, but how could it be? The doctor said the pathologists were 95 percent sure, but because I was breastfeeding at the time of the biopsy, the milk may have mixed with the tissue sample so they weren't 100 percent sure and were working on it.

"So maybe it's not cancer, then," I said.

He stood up. "I'll give you some time to think about this." Then he left the room.

Where did he go? To grab a coffee? To meet a patient who *didn't* have cancer? My life had just divided in two, so where the hell was he off to? I looked at the two people still there with me.

"I feel like this is a death sentence," I blurted out.

I have to give credit to my husband and my mother: They were both rock solid.

Greg said, "You'll be fine." I think he and my mom were holding my hands, but to be honest, I can't quite remember.

My mother was trembling. "Alana, we will fight this thing. You are going to fight this."

I was frozen. I felt like the walls and the ceiling were caving in on me, and there was nothing I could do to stop it from happening.

Doctor 3 returned and sat down. "I can perform a lumpectomy," he said, explaining that he would surgically remove the lump and the surrounding tissue under local anesthetic. "It's a fairly common procedure. I would love to get you in for surgery next week, but I'm going on vacation, and this is one of those situations where we need to 'hurry up and wait.'"

What? What did he just say?

"I can book you in for surgery on October 19."

It was September 15. How was I supposed to wait more than a month with this *thing* growing inside me?

My mother, who had been silent while he'd been talking, leapt into action. "Should we take Alana to a bigger cancer center? Maybe they'd be faster? What about the Juravinski Centre in Hamilton?" She was referring to the Juravinski Cancer Centre, or JCC, a large treatment facility located nearby in Hamilton, Ontario.

"Studies show that we have good luck in smaller, local hospitals," Doctor 3 responded.

Good luck? Good *luck*?

"This is my daughter we're talking about," Mom said. "We want the best treatment available."

Doctor 3 again replied that he was sure he could successfully perform this surgery.

Mom and I looked at each other. Everyone needs a vacation, I understood that. I wanted to go on vacation at that moment, too. In fact, I wanted to get the hell out of that office and escape from the nightmare I was in, but I couldn't. I had a cancerous tumor growing inside me. I couldn't wait for a surgeon to come back from his vacation to get it removed. I knew my family was thinking the exact same thing.

We left the office and walked towards the elevator. The ride down felt like I was sinking into a new and horrible world. I had cancer. I couldn't step back over that threshold into before. My life before cancer was over.

$\mathcal{P}$

Dead silence in the car on the way home. My mom gave me a huge hug when she left us in the parking lot, and surprisingly she kept it together, so I tried to keep it together for her as well. I was shaking, though. I was in shock. Greg had left work to come to the appointment with me, so before we started driving, he phoned his boss and told him that he wasn't coming back that afternoon. Although I heard only one side of the conversation, and it was brief, I could imagine exactly what his boss had said. It was just that kind of conversation. "Oh, no! The results were positive? I'm so sorry. Let us know if we can help. Please tell her we are praying for her and thinking of her."

I started thinking about what this world would be like without me. Cars flickered past me, filled with people going about their lives. They would still be there when I was gone.

I think Greg knew that I didn't want to talk, and he allowed me that time to just think. He kept looking over at me, but I stared straight ahead. I know he was genuinely worried, but what could he do to help? It was a long ride, and as I stared blankly out the window, I started thinking about what this world would be like without me. Cars flickered past me, filled with people going about their lives. They would still be there when I was gone.

When we arrived home, the kids were waiting to greet us. The baby-sitter knew full well from our faces what had taken place. No words were necessary. I went to our bedroom, closed the door and cried. I didn't want to see anyone, didn't want to talk to anyone, didn't want to be around anyone, because what could I possibly say? I had cancer. I wished that I could ignore it and it would all go away, but I knew that wouldn't happen. I knew that my mother would tell my father and grandmother, and my sister and brother. Greg would tell his family.

I did have one friend who called to find out how things went, a colleague from work, Melanie. When she asked me, I started crying and couldn't speak. But I didn't have to. "I'm so sorry," she said, and I heard her start to cry as well. Then our wordless conversation ended.

That evening was rough, probably the roughest night I've had. The more distraught I became, the more sadness set in. The one emotion that kept rising to the surface, though, was anger, and I think this was my defense mechanism: "I'll be damned if I'm going to let this take over my life!"

I kept asking myself questions.

Why?

Why did this happen to me?

What did I do to deserve this?

Why did I not find this earlier?

And of course, why can't I make this go away?

Chapter 5

POSITIVE THOUGHTS, DAMN IT!

*T**he next morning* my father appeared unannounced at my house. I hadn't seen him since the official diagnosis.

"Oh, Dad, please don't," I said as he wiped tears away. I motioned for him to come in. He did and started to take off his shoes while I went to get him a tissue from the bathroom. We aren't real huggy types—never have been. When I got back, he was still standing by the front door.

"Thank you," he said. He took the tissue and asked, "Where are the kids?" even as his eyes started to well up again.

"You can't do this, you know," I said.

"I'm sorry, Alana, I'm just scared."

"I know, Dad. So am I. But I can't keep crying about this, it's not going to help anything. Come in the kitchen. I'm going to make us some coffee."

"That sounds good. I didn't sleep much last night. I'm sorry," he said again.

"Don't worry. Neither did I."

We got our coffee and sat on the couch and sipped it. I spent the rest of the visit reassuring Dad that everything would be okay, even though I wasn't so sure myself. I was discovering that one of the strange side effects of getting diagnosed with cancer is having to comfort those around you who are distraught because of your diagnosis. When he left, I closed the door behind him and slumped against it. I was exhausted. The negativity simply had to stop. It was draining me, and I had to find a way to be positive. I had to start believing in the power of positive thinking. I was going to be a cancer survivor, I told myself. I was going to grow old and enjoy watching my children grow up.

I had to find a way to be positive. I had to start believing in the power of positive thinking. I was going to be a cancer survivor, I told myself. I was going to grow old and enjoy watching my children grow up.

I went back to the kitchen, found an elastic band and put it around my wrist. Every time I thought something negative, I would snap it, hard. By the time a week had passed, there were far fewer anxious and overwhelming moments. Soon the elastic band came off. I remained positive and driven, focusing less on "poor me" and more on "kicking cancer's ass." I had to fight. I had to stay strong. No one else was going to wage this battle for me. I turned on my warrior mode. I wanted to enter into this war guns blazing.

I phoned my mammogram technician.

It was as if she had been waiting for me to call. "I'm sorry. I couldn't say anything," she said, revealing what I'd suspected—that she had seen something. "Can I visit you?"

"Of course!" I said.

That night we talked over a bottle of wine, discussing everything: what I should expect; what a lumpectomy means; what a mastectomy means; what types of breast cancer there are; what types of treatments are available. When she mentioned the word *chemotherapy*, I froze. I ran my hand through my hair. I would likely lose it, I realized. *I am so naive*, I thought. I felt blindsided, but before I could even process that, she told me that the technician who had performed my ultrasound had battled breast cancer, too, and I was drawn out of my own tragedy into someone else's.

"She was diagnosed in her thirties, just like you."

"I knew I heard something extra in her voice during my appointment. How awful. It must have been so fresh in her mind."

"She felt bad, but she couldn't say anything, either."

The more we talked, the more I came to understand that I was my biggest advocate: I was one single patient, while each of my doctors had many patients. No one cared about my health more than I did. I decided then that I would read and learn everything there was to know about breast cancer. The more information I had, the better off I'd be.

After our visit, I began to ask for advice from anyone I knew who had a medical background. I bought a notebook and began writing everything down, documenting all of my phone calls and the information I gathered. I did the same thing at all of my appointments. Doing that empowered me, made me feel that I was actually doing something to beat the cancer. The more I did, the more positive I felt. I decided that I wanted around me only those people who were going to be as strong as I was trying so hard to be. An incredible energy came over me—positive energy. That was what I needed most, and I had to put that idea out there. I started drafting an e-mail.

Hello, everyone,

I'm writing to let you know about some bad news we received this week. The only reason I'm e-mailing is because right now I'm finding it really hard to talk about it, so this seemed the best way to let you know directly from me. On Wednesday, after much testing, I was diagnosed with breast

cancer. It's difficult for me to even write that word, because doing that
acknowledges that it's not just a bad dream, that I have to deal with it,
that I have to be strong. . . .

The underlying message was clear: Don't come over if you're going to
cry at my door.

ℰ

Before Doctor 3 had gone on his vacation, he referred me for a chest X-ray
and ultrasound. Erin came with me because I didn't want her to feel left
out. Plus there were simple logistics to deal with: Greg was working and I
needed my mom to watch the kids.

Again the technicians didn't say much, but I knew not to expect any
answers from them, so I stopped asking questions. I knew what the tests
were for: to see if the cancer had spread. After a lot of reading I was aware
that if it had spread to my other organs, it wouldn't be good. Most likely
Stage 4. Most likely fatal. I simply lay there on the cold table, again draped
in one of those blue hospital gowns, until they were done with my body.
That was how I had begun to think of it—as a body, a vessel, distancing
myself from it, especially my breasts. I didn't want to touch them or look at
them. The act of separation was already beginning.

Afterwards, I made arrangements to pick up the films to bring with
me on appointments—those from both the X-ray and the ultrasound, as
well as both mammograms. I felt that if I went equipped with my trusty
notebook and as much information as possible, the doctors would provide
me with even more information in return. They'd know how serious I was.

I had to meet with another surgeon to see if I could get my lumpectomy
bumped up to an earlier date. I couldn't wait until Doctor 3 came back from
vacation. Doctor 5 was a surgeon from a neighboring city who came highly
recommended by my mom. She was the person Mom dealt with when she
had her biopsy scare. We didn't have an abundance of surgeons in our area
who dealt with breast cancer, but I'd asked a few other people about her

as well, and everyone had good things to say, including my family doctor. I thought, *Maybe a vacation won't be more important to her than my health.* And she was a woman.

"She's extremely knowledgeable and personable," Mom had told me. And it turned out she was all those things. But she couldn't get me into surgery any earlier. In fact, she wouldn't be able to operate on me until a week *later* than Doctor 3, on November 2. I walked out of her office, carrying my stack of files and scans, feeling deflated. More than that, in fact, helpless. How could I wait that long?

I had dinner with friends that night. One of them was a nurse at the local hospital. I told her everything that was going on—not surprising since my cancer seemed to be the topic of every single conversation I had with people. I couldn't escape it even when I tried. She asked me if I'd been sent for a bone scan.

"Why a bone scan?" I asked.

"Your oncologist is likely going to want you to have one done. Rather than wait, you should try to have it done now so nothing gets pushed back because they're waiting for more test results," she said.

The next day I was on a mission. I called my family doctor's office and asked if I could see him that day—surely he would refer me for a scan right away. He wasn't working that particular day, so another doctor was filling in for him. The receptionist told me I could come by if I wanted, so I packed up the kids—stroller, diaper bag, toys, snacks and all—and headed over.

The kids were cranky before we even got there. Rudy was tired, fidgety and hungry for more than snacks. When wasn't he hungry, though? Charley was overdue for her nap and got tired of sitting around. We were called in after about an hour. Once inside an exam room, we waited another ten minutes before the doctor came in. I got right to the point. "I want a bone scan," I said. I think I was so abrupt I alarmed him.

"Why?"

"I have cancer. I've had a mammogram. I've had an ultrasound. I'm going for a lumpectomy. My oncologist might want me to get a bone scan. Please refer me for one."

"Why don't you wait and see if your oncologist wants you to have one?"

"I don't want to wait. I want one done now."

He tried to stay calm, because it obviously appeared to him that I *wasn't* calm, and the kids were climbing all over me.

"You seem stressed," he said. "Maybe I can refer you to talk to someone."

In my mind I started screaming at him. Talk to someone? Like who? A therapist? A psychologist? None of those people would help with my cancer. He had to be kidding. I was on the verge of tears, and by that point, the kids were downright miserable. "Listen, we're not leaving this office until you write up a requisition for a bone scan. Simple." So much for my mother's lesson about being polite.

I don't know if it was me or the kids he didn't want to deal with anymore, but he left the office and came back with a slip of paper. The bone scan was performed later that week. In the end, my chest X-ray, ultrasound and bone scan results all came in clear—the cancer hadn't spread to my lungs, my liver or any other organs in my abdominal area. For the first time, I had information that made me think there might be some hope. But I had to make a decision. Option 1: surgery on October 19 with Doctor 3, or Option 2: surgery on November 2 with Doctor 5, whom I felt comfortable and confident with.

It was already Thursday, September 30. After much debate with myself, I decided to go with Doctor 3. Only because the surgery would be earlier.

The next day, on October 1, the phone rang. I picked up reluctantly. I didn't know who was calling, and I didn't always feel up to talking about what was going on.

"Hey, Alana, it's Monica. How are things going? How are you holding up?"

I was relieved when I realized who it was. I'd met Monica when our kids were taking gymnastics together, and we'd instantly connected. "Not bad. I'm kind of frustrated with how long I have to wait for things." I explained what had happened with the two surgeons.

"Totally understand."

I knew she did—Monica was also a doctor.

"Would you like me to try to get you into Juravinski to see a surgeon there?"

I don't know if I even let her finish her sentence. "I'm not sure. Isn't it a big hospital? I don't want to be just a number." I paused. "I guess it would be worth a shot to see if I can get in earlier."

"Let me see what I can do. I can get back to you shortly."

I immediately had a glimmer of hope. After all, the two doctors I'd seen locally couldn't get me in for surgery before October 19, so the idea I'd get in earlier anywhere else had seemed impossible. But would I get lost in the crowd at a larger center? Would I end up being just a number, so to speak? Would the care be worse rather than better, if that were the case?

"Sure," I said. It was the best decision I ever made.

Chapter 6

SQUEAKY WHEEL

It became increasingly obvious to me that in our health care system, and indeed in life in general, the more you push, the more you get. It didn't hurt to know people, either. Half an hour after I spoke with Monica, the phone rang. She got me in! I had an appointment with a surgeon at the JCC at one-thirty that very afternoon.

It was ten-thirty in the morning. I began to scramble to find a babysitter, and luckily Greg's boss's wife, Susanne, who lived right down the road, was able to come over to watch the kids for me. I was so grateful. I still needed to get lunch prepped for the kids, get myself dressed, organize and assemble the files that I wanted to bring along, and call my mother to arrange to meet somewhere. I also had to get myself ready psychologically for this next step. What would this surgeon say? Would she be any different from any of the doctors I had already seen? And of more immediate concern, when would she be able to operate on me?

I managed to get my act together, and Mom and I made it to JCC in time. Any anxieties I had of being just a number vanished the moment my mother and I walked into the center. What a beautiful, welcoming building. Not only was it new, the light that emanated from within was radiant. I had been expecting a somber and melancholy place, but while it was obvious it was a cancer center because of the number of women with scarves on their heads, undoubtedly a telltale sign that they had lost their hair from chemotherapy, it was the most upbeat hospital lobby I'd ever seen, with smiling people bustling about. I have to admit I was taken aback by the sheer number of people I saw. And people I wouldn't have looked at twice on the street, whom I wouldn't have registered in any way as cancer patients, were clearly there for one reason: They had cancer, too, and there were so many of them—*of us*, I thought after a moment, realizing I wasn't alone.

We went to the doctor's office, where we had to sit only briefly in the waiting room before being shown into an office. Everyone we encountered was so friendly and welcoming, they made me feel they genuinely cared.

Doctor 6 walked in. She was young, kind and drop-dead gorgeous. We started talking and discovered that we lived less than ten kilometers away from each other. I couldn't help but think it was a sign. Most important, she knew what she was talking about. She examined me carefully, and while I was half hoping she would tell me that the other doctors had it all wrong, she unfortunately confirmed what they'd said.

"The lump feels like it's approximately two centimeters big, and I think one of your lymph nodes is enlarged."

When it came to surgery dates, the news wasn't good, either. For some bizarre reason I'd envisioned that she'd have an open schedule the following week, but she didn't have anything available till mid-November. Of course she didn't. She was a top doctor in a major cancer center. Why wouldn't she be booked solid? That was when I started begging.

"I really want you to do the surgery, I need you to do this for me, but I don't want to wait. Please, can't you fit me in sooner?"

"I'll try to find some available operating room time and will see if I can squeeze you in. But I won't be able to give you an answer right away."

I saw compassion in her eyes, something I hadn't seen yet in a doctor. At least not to that extent. "Please," I said.

"I'll see what I can do." She smiled sympathetically. "My nurse will call you Monday morning."

$\mathcal{P}$

Sometimes, if you want something badly enough, it will happen. At least that's what I kept hoping. I wanted Doctor 6, and I wanted the surgery done as soon as possible. I spent all weekend with my fingers crossed. I tried to keep busy. I took Charley to gymnastics, and we went to dinner at my mom's on Saturday night. On Sunday I threw myself into some much-needed yard work. I also continued to wean Rudy. After the diagnosis, I had been told I'd have to stop breastfeeding. This was a bitter moment for me. While I'd decided three weeks previously that it was time to start the process, the decision wasn't in my hands any longer. I felt pangs of guilt and worried that he would be missing out on health benefits. But I had no choice in the matter. It was happening whether I wanted it to or not.

All weekend, I couldn't stop thinking about the surgery. On Monday I spent the morning waiting for the call Doctor 6 had promised. Nothing. In the afternoon the phone finally rang. My surgeon had traded operating room time with another doctor, and I was scheduled for surgery on October 12, a full week before the earliest surgery I'd been able to get before. I couldn't believe it! She was my angel, a miracle worker, and all my efforts had paid off! Was it because we lived so close to each other? Was it because I had begged? Was it because she was just a great human being with compassion? No matter what the reason, I was ecstatic.

I went into overdrive—there were so many more appointments I had to fit in before my surgery.

I'd never had surgery before—the most I'd had were my wisdom teeth out in the dentist's office—so I went to my first preoperative appointment.

The nurses explained what I had to do before the surgery and what was about to happen: I couldn't have anything to eat or drink after midnight; I had to check in at the front desk upon arrival; avoid exercise for two to three weeks after; and take Tylenol 3 as needed for the pain, but definitely for the next few days after surgery, as they'd be the worst.

Oddly, I didn't feel scared, just nervous about the anesthetic. I'd heard horror stories about people not waking up because of it, and I was afraid I might be one of those people. But again, what choice did I have in the matter?

The next appointment was for a breast MRI. This time a technician prepped a syringe and injected a radioactive dye into a vein in my right hand. I watched as the syringe was emptied into me so the dye could begin to mix with my blood. The dye was clear. In fact, it looked like saline, but it was far from it. This stuff would course through my veins and help the technicians find any more cancer in my body. I thought that I would feel it in some way—I mean, after all, it was radioactive. But I felt nothing. My understanding was that if the tumor was a cyst, blood wouldn't flow into it, but if it was cancer, blood would flow into it to feed it. After the dye had been given a chance to make its way through my system, I was asked to take off all my clothing above the waist and drape myself in a hospital gown with the ties at the front. By then, my breasts had already been seen by so many people that the gown seemed pointless. I lay facedown on the MRI table, with my breasts suspended in two slots. We were a team of three: me, a technician in the room with me who assisted with directions and suggestions and who consulted with a second technician in an adjoining room, who apparently was looking at computer images of my breasts to make sure everything was in clear view. It took me a couple of minutes to adjust myself so they could get the best picture possible.

The technicians were great, and as they worked, I tried to make small talk. Maybe that was a stall tactic on my part—if I kept them talking about other things, they wouldn't be able to tell me bad news. Or maybe it was exactly the opposite: If I talked with them enough and managed to get them to feel sympathetic towards me, they would tell me everything they knew. They told me that when they first got the machines at the hospital, they practiced on each other to achieve the best comfort level for patients, since the position was painful for many. They even told me how they'd performed a breast MRI on another colleague and found a four-centimeter lump in her breast that previously had gone undetected. That amazed me. I was naive enough to think that if you worked in the medical profession, you would somehow know more about the human body and would be able to find abnormalities like that in your own body way before they got to that stage.

I found myself quite comfortable lying in the MRI machine. My head was resting on its side, and I felt as though I was ready to take a nap. I didn't experience any of the claustrophobia some people talk about. I could easily have fallen asleep if it hadn't been for the loud clicking sound the machine made. I even felt brave enough to venture *the* question. "Do you see anything unusual?"

No response.

I held my breath.

"I can't see anything."

I exhaled. Of course, even as I did so, I knew that didn't mean there wasn't anything there.

Chapter 7

WILL I WAKE UP AGAIN?

ℐ

The day of the surgery, I woke up at five A.M. It was pitch black out, dead quiet, and I was wired. I had to be at the hospital at 7:15 A.M., even though the operation wasn't until ten. My mother had slept over the night before. She'd volunteered to come over again to watch the kids while I had surgery. I thought about her while I rolled out of bed. How would I feel if one of my children was going to be operated on? I couldn't imagine she'd had an easy night—not that she'd ever say anything.

Everyone was asleep, so I quietly moved about getting ready. Our kids were usually light sleepers—mornings at our house were hectic so it was sometimes difficult to keep them from waking up. About a half hour before we had to leave, I crept back into the bedroom to wake Greg up, and by the time I got back to the kitchen, Mom was there. I did a few more things while she hung out with me and then with Greg when he came out to grab breakfast, and thankfully the kids slept through it all.

Greg drove to the hospital. We didn't talk much. My mind was left to drift in every direction possible. Would I wake up from the anesthetic? Would they find more cancer when they went in there? Would it hurt afterwards? For how long? The questions kept coming, and I knew that depending on the outcome of this surgery, my life could go in two different directions once again.

We pulled into the parking lot, and the hospital was already buzzing, despite the early hour. In the admitting department I filled out what seemed like a huge stack of paperwork (I felt as though I was signing my life away). Next we headed up to the nuclear medicine department to meet my surgeon. When we got there, I stopped in front of the doors. The nuclear symbols on them loomed large: corrosive, explosive, flammable. Nothing could have felt less inviting, but through the doors I went, despite all my inhibitions.

Inside, I found myself in a large open room filled with big machines, where a nurse asked me to disrobe and lie on a metal table in the center of the room. I felt as though I was about to take part in a strange experiment, which in a sense I was. My surgeon, Doctor 6, came in and I felt a bit better. Something about her calm and confident demeanor relaxed me, as much as I could relax given the situation. *Angel*, I kept thinking. *She's my angel. She's got this.*

"How are you doing?" she asked.

"Okay." What else could I say? But I appreciated her asking.

She nodded and turned around. When she turned back, she held a long, slender syringe filled with a blue liquid. My blood pressure ratcheted up. "I'm going to inject radioactive dye into your nipple area," she explained, and her eyes drifted away from mine to focus on my chest. I steeled myself for the inevitable pain. I was surprised, though. It didn't hurt as much as I thought it would. Maybe all of those months of breastfeeding Rudy had made my nipples super tough.

"The dye will make its way into your lymph nodes," she said. "The whole point of this is to identify where your sentinel lymph nodes, the nodes that cancer is most likely to spread to first, are. During surgery, I'll identify those sentinel nodes and take out three or four of them to check if they're cancerous. Those first few nodes are like a first line of defense. The cancer has to get through those before it can travel farther."

I watched the level in the syringe drop as she talked. I thought about the blue dye silently creeping into my sentinel nodes. I imagined those nodes as border security and U.S. customs agents. How many were on the front line of defense? If the cancer was able to get past them, where would it go after that? What corner of my body would it sneak into?

"If those nodes are cancerous, I'll remove the remaining nodes. All of them. If cancer hasn't spread to the sentinel nodes, it's unlikely it will have gone any farther, so your lymph nodes will stay intact."

She pushed the dye into me. After that, I had to wait another two hours. I walked every hallway of that hospital several times. I was so nervous. I tried to memorize my surroundings in an odd sort of memory game, but that didn't help. Neither did reading magazines in the lobby. While I paced, Greg ate. It was probably his way of dealing with the anxiety. He kept checking in, asking if I wanted anything or if he could help, but there was nothing he could do. I don't know if I expected him to follow the same protocol I had to—not eating before surgery—but watching him eat was driving me crazy. I was starving and couldn't sit still.

I called my mother to update her. "Hi, Mom." I tried to picture myself as a brave warrior.

"Hi. What's happening?" She sounded almost as nervous as I was.

I told her about the dye, and that the surgery was about forty-five minutes away. "Can I talk to the kids?" I asked. I was trying to keep my voice steady, but it had fallen off to a shaky whisper.

I heard her calling, "Charley, Mommy is on the phone." Then Charley's little voice sounded in my ear.

"Hi, Mommy."

"Hi, Charley. Are you having a good morning? Are you having fun with Babcia?" *Babcia* is Polish for grandmother.

"Mommy, I love you," Charley said, and then she was gone. I was glad she was happy, but I admit I wanted her to miss me. My little girl was okay without me. She didn't need me. I looked at all the sick people around me. Was I going to be like them? Was that already me? Did I suddenly have a time stamp on my life? Would I make it out of this alive? Would Charley and Rudy have to live their lives without their mom? What was happening seemed surreal, a bizarre dream. It hadn't turned into a nightmare yet, because I didn't feel sick, but it certainly wasn't a good dream. I hung up the phone and started pacing again.

At nine A.M., I was called in to get ready for surgery.

"Here we go," I said to Greg as I headed over to the nurse who called my name.

"Relax, you will be fine. You're in good hands," he reminded me.

And off I went with the nurse to a preop area. Greg would be able to come in after I was prepped. I thought everything would be sterile and cold, but it was good to discover that wasn't the case. I was given a snug blue gown to change into, and there were nice warm little bootees for my feet. Then I got to hang out in a comfortable leather lounge chair while a nurse started my IV. She said I had little veins and it might take a couple of tries, but I didn't even feel a pinch and the line was in, taped and ready to go. I also received an injection of heparin in my thigh to prevent blood clots—apparently a standard pre-surgery procedure.

"I think they mentioned that to me in the preop appointment, but there was so much information that day, it all became somewhat of a blur," I said to the nurse in a rush. I think I was babbling.

She smiled. "It's a lot to take in."

That needle didn't hurt, either, other than a tiny pinch. When she was done, she covered me with a warm blanket and let Greg come and sit with me.

"Are you ready for this?" he asked.

"Ready as I'll ever be," I said, trying to play it cool, even though I was terrified I wouldn't wake up after surgery. "Will you keep my mom posted?"

"Yes, I'll tell her everything that happens." I felt scared. I didn't know what else to say. Obviously Greg didn't, either.

Right before surgery, Doctor 6 showed up. She asked me which breast she was going to operate on. She knew it was the left breast, I knew it was the left breast, but it was protocol to ask. After we both verified verbally that it was actually the left breast, she wrote her initial on it with a felt-tipped pen. (Artwork on my body! That was a first.) The marker on my skin tickled. You'd think I would have started laughing, but as Doctor 6 leaned over me, I noticed that her surgical cap was pale pink and that it was covered in a pale pink ribbon design. I choked up. Everything became real. This wasn't a dream. It wasn't just any surgery I was going in for. This was about *breast cancer*. I had to take a minute before I gave Greg a kiss and could say good-bye to him.

I'd expected to be wheeled to the operating room and lifted up onto the table—that was the way I'd seen it done in the movies. Instead, I set off with the nurse on what seemed like the longest walk of my life. And when we arrived in the operating room, I was simply asked to get up onto the table. By then I was shaking uncontrollably. I kept looking around the room, and the more I looked, the more nervous I became. Everything was so unwelcoming and high tech: giant fluorescent lights hanging from the ceiling, metal trays with masses of surgical tools, whiteboards with code words I couldn't decipher. There were no warm and fuzzy decorations. There were no cute drawings by previous patients the way there were elsewhere. There were no chatty discussions.

There were so many people—three nurses, an anesthesiologist, and the surgeon and her resident. To my mind, if the situation involved so many people, it must be way more serious than I'd been thinking. I mean, I knew it was serious, but this amount of attention was freaking me out. Everyone swarmed about, busily prepping for surgery, while I lay on the table shaking, those giant lights blinding me. I felt like a specimen, pinned, silent and scared. One of the nurses put a warm blanket over me, which helped.

Eventually Doctor 6 came over to me to explain how the radioactive injection they'd given me earlier would work. She pointed at an instrument, saying, "That's my *Star Wars* machine," and waved a wand over my breast and armpit area. The wand made noises that did sound like something from the *Star Wars* movies. "I'll use this to pinpoint exactly where your sentinel lymph nodes are," she said. "That's how I'll know which ones to take out." She sounded so confident. This would be easy. She knew what she was doing.

The anesthesiologist put a mask over my face, asked me to breathe deeply, Doctor 6 said, "Here comes the good stuff," and that is the last thing I remember.

Chapter 8

MISSING PIECES

I *woke up in* the recovery room two hours later. Greg's face was the first I saw. I recall him saying I was awake, and I kept hearing muffled voices, so I'm sure he was chatting with the nurses, but I was so out of it I had no idea what was being said and just wanted to fall back asleep again. I felt lethargic and very confused. Apparently Doctor 6 came to speak with me after the surgery, but I have no recollection of that at all. It was the strangest feeling, not knowing exactly what had happened during two hours of my life, although it definitely ranks up there as one of the best sleeps I've ever had. Luckily, Greg was able to tell me what she said.

The lump was removed, and it measured 2.9 centimeters. I later found out that 3 centimeters would have possibly meant a different stage in my cancer diagnosis, so that 1 millimeter was very important. Doctor 6 also removed four lymph nodes. Of those, only one seemed a little larger than normal—that was the one that had shown up on my MRI. I'd brought that MRI scan to JCC. When I'd first seen her, Doctor 6 had told me that a patient's scans are only as good as the person who reads them. So I'd begun getting every single scan burned onto individual disks, which I carried around with me. It seemed logical that since the doctors and nurses at JCC work with cancer all the time, they look at any images in addition to the original radiologists. As it turned out, the two radiologists who looked at my MRI came up with two slightly different results. Both agreed, though, that one of the sentinel nodes was enlarged, but they differed on whether this meant cancer for sure.

✑

Greg reported that Doctor 6 removed the enlarged node and three other nodes, and sent them all for a frozen section while I was on the operating table, which meant those nodes were flash frozen, then cut open to see if there was any cancer inside. Even though I was sort of out of it, I remembered that I had signed a waiver before surgery saying that if more cancer was found, an axillary dissection to remove all of my lymph nodes could be done. "Thankfully," Greg assured me, "no visible cancer was found."

The main recovery room was quite hectic, so after about half an hour, I was moved to a quieter room with fewer nurses and machines. "Once you're able to get up and use the washroom on your own and we check your incision and change the dressing one last time to make sure everything is good, we can release you," a nurse told us. Before they let me go, though, a nurse showed me how to change the dressing myself. I found I couldn't look at the incision. I wasn't ready to see what they had done to me.

About two hours after I came out of surgery, the nurse officially released me and we got ready to leave the hospital. I was tired, but felt surprisingly good. My chest was sore, but didn't hurt as much as I'd expected. Before we left the room there was something I needed to do. How much of me was missing? I wondered. I finally reached up to feel it. I was bandaged so well there was no movement at all in my breast area, which I realized helped tremendously, but I couldn't tell how big a piece was gone.

Greg wheeled me out. When we got to the doorway of the hospital, I said, "Stop here. I can walk the rest of the way." I sounded so determined that he didn't try to change my mind. I walked the entire way to the car, not because I wanted to be a hero, but because I felt fine. On the way home, we picked up the Tylenol 3 with codeine that had been prescribed for pain, just in case.

I was so relieved when we finally got home. Mom smiled from ear to ear when she saw me and insisted I rest on the couch. The kids were watching TV, so I gently snuggled up next to them and tried to relax while Greg went outside to do some yard work. I lounged around for the rest of the day, but by the time Mom was making dinner, I was up for playing with the kids.

"You're sure you're okay?" Mom asked.

"I'm fine," I assured her, and physically speaking I *was*. I didn't need the prescription we'd gotten—Extra Strength Tylenol ended up being enough to alleviate any discomfort I had. I even slept well that night. I was fine on another level, too. I was so glad that a big step of the journey was over and done with. I was alive. And although I had much more of a battle ahead of me, I felt motivated; I felt like I had my boxing gloves on, ready for the next stage in this war.

All the week after the surgery, my mom stayed with Greg and me, helping out as much as she could. One of my friends, Adriana, brought delicious homemade Italian meals over, and had ever since I was first diagnosed. I tried to do as much as I used to, but found I couldn't. Rudy was eight months old and a hefty twenty-five pounds. I wasn't able to lift him into his crib, get him into his high chair, put him on the changing table to change his diaper, or even give him a bottle. It ripped my heart out. In what seemed like an instant, I wasn't able to hold my baby or care for him the way I used to.

I changed Rudy, but on the carpet in his room. I fed him his bottles, but he crawled up onto a pillow on my lap as I sat on the carpet leaning against the couch. And his new bed became a mattress on the floor. My eight-month-old son was sleeping on a mattress on the floor!

My bandages stayed on for the first few days; then I removed them. I wasn't that sore anymore and the doctor had said it would be all right. Plus, having the bandages off made things much easier—I didn't need to be so careful keeping them dry when I was showering. I left the surgical tape on the incisions for a couple of weeks, and after that it peeled off without any problems.

My relationship with my body changed. When I used to get out of the shower, the first thing I would do was slather myself with lotion. I still used lotion, but as I stood in front of the mirror, I realized that I'd been skipping the breast area entirely, even before the surgery. I didn't even refer to them as "my breasts" anymore.

My breasts. They were nice, once. My bra size was 32C. My breasts weren't big enough to look like they didn't fit my body type, but I was far from flat-chested. I didn't wear cleavage-showing tops (I was a bit conservative that way). But on more than one occasion I noticed men looking at them. I wasn't offended. I was flattered, to be honest. I felt sexy. I felt strong. They made me feel like I was a woman. I did not want cancer to rip from my body the two things that made me feel very much like a woman: my breasts and my long hair.

> My relationship with my body changed. . . . I did not want cancer to rip from my body the two things that made me feel very much like a woman: my breasts and my long hair.

When I first found the lump, I felt it at least twenty times a day, wishing each time that it wouldn't be there anymore, each time not believing that it *was* there. After I was officially diagnosed, I was afraid of it. Afraid if I touched it, that would make it spread; afraid that the next time I touched it, it would be bigger. After the surgery, not only the lump was gone, but part of my breast was gone, too. When I finally had the nerve to look, there was a dent. It was as if a golf-ball-sized piece had been taken out, and the remaining parts sewed back together without filling the void first. Nothing was in its proper place anymore, and it simply looked deformed. If a mastectomy was in my future, my entire breast would no longer be a part of the body I cherished and loved, would no longer define my womanhood.

Chapter 9

BAD NEWS

I had to wait three anxious weeks after the lumpectomy surgery to meet with my surgeon, Doctor 6, to get the results of the pathology tests.

"The good news is that the margins of the tumor were clear, meaning that when I removed the lump, I got all of it," she explained.

"That's great!" I said. For a fleeting moment I felt like things were going my way, but I realized she had more to say.

"The bad news is that one of the four lymph nodes I removed has tested positive for cancer. A small section contained cancer cells—a very small section, 2.2 millimeters—but they were there nonetheless."

I started to feel familiar waves of panic. Doctor 6 kept talking, and I struggled to pay attention. I knew I wasn't the only one. Greg was there with me, struggling, too. Doctor 6 had to be struggling as well. She lived so close to me. We knew some of the same people. She was young. She empathized—I could see that. I empathized with her—how horrible it must be to pass on such bad news.

"When deciding what stage a woman's cancer is at, a few things come into play," she said. "The size of the tumor, if any lymph nodes are positive, as well as the grade of the tumor, which indicates how fast and aggressively the cancer cells are growing. The grade of a tumor is numbered one, two or three, with one being the least aggressive and three being the most aggressive." She paused. "Your tumor is grade three."

I stared at her, speechless. Greg squeezed my hand. Normally that would make me feel good. Loved. But in the face of such devastating news, I was numb. What could anyone do that was going to comfort me or help me?

"Your cancer is categorized as Stage 2B and also triple negative, which means your particular cancer cells are not receptive to estrogen, progesterone or HER2/neu."

Was it my imagination or had her voice wavered? How on earth could anything be worse than what she'd already told me?

"What does that mean?" I managed to ask.

"Many women with triple negative breast cancer will go on to test positive for the BRCA1 or BRCA2 mutation," she said, explaining that if I tested positive, that could result in an increased risk of breast cancer for members of my family—Charley, my mother, my sister, my nieces. The men in my life weren't immune, either. The risk to them was much lower, but it was there. I thought of my children. That embarrassment I'd been feeling turned into shame and guilt. It would be my fault if my daughter got breast cancer one day. It would be my fault if my son were one of those men affected. I was mortified.

Doctor 6's words drifted into my consciousness, plus other words that I associated with cancer. Chemotherapy. Mastectomy. Radiation. Referrals to other doctors. I tried to focus. The oncologist had to decide, she said, but once the lymph nodes were involved, chemotherapy was usually part of the treatment, and perhaps radiation, in order to kill the cancer cells. I think she said I'd have to meet with both an oncologist and a radiologist to find out for sure. I slumped in my chair. Charley and Rudy. I'd never imagined that stupid lump would have anything to do with them. This wasn't just *my* disease anymore. Doctor 6's words bounced around in my head till they became all confused. It was too much to handle.

◦

Back home, I tried to keep busy. I wrote another e-mail—after all, I'd committed to letting people know how things were going. And I wanted everyone to think I was fine, that I was holding my shit together. But I was discovering just how deceptive appearances could be.

> *Hello, everyone,*
>
> *I apologize for the informality of an e-mail, but this seemed to be the best way to get information out to everyone about the pathology results and prognosis.*
>
> *First things first: The tumor is out! She got it all! One of the four lymph nodes removed contained a very small cancerous growth, but since the others were clear, it's unlikely there's any more cancer. My other scans were okay, so, in essence, I'm cancer-free at the moment!*
>
> *Now I'm waiting for an appointment with an oncologist. I'll probably end up having to have a bunch of chemo appointments. That means I'll be inviting anyone who wants to keep me company for the day to call in sick to work—maybe we could even squeeze in some shopping!*
>
> *Very likely I'll be bald in time for Christmas and Santa, but if I'm a good girl, perhaps he'll bring me something to keep my head warm!!!*
>
> *Thanks to everyone for the cards, phone calls, cookies and dinner plans. We appreciate everything and are going to kick this thing in the butt!*

I cried as I typed that e-mail. I was scared. I didn't want to be going through this. I didn't want to lose my hair. I didn't want to die. It wasn't fair, and I was angry. I cried afterwards, when I was alone. I paced up and down; I punched the wall. I was crumbling inside, but I didn't want anyone, especially my parents or my children, to know how truly frightened I was. They were afraid themselves, and if they knew how I felt, it would be so difficult for them. *This is my fault*, I thought.

Part Two

FIRST STEPS

Chapter 10

ONCOLOGY LOGIC

L *ucky. I wasn't* exactly feeling like I was leading a charmed existence, but genetic testing is expensive, and I qualified to have it done at no charge, since I was under thirty-five years of age when I was diagnosed. And I'd get the results relatively soon—in approximately eight weeks.

I decided to take two of the most important women in my life, my mother and my sister, to my appointment with the genetics counselor. If the results were positive, it would affect them first. I tried to explain the implications to Erin.

"If the test comes back positive, that could mean that you and Natalie are at risk." Natalie, Erin's daughter, was only six.

"I'm not sure I'd want to know," she said. "Or if I'd want to know about

Natalie, either. How would that change our lives? How we do things? How we think of the future?"

I thought about what she said. She had a point. I didn't know what the next step would be for me or if I'd want to know about my own kids. Would we live in fear? Would changing anything we did affect the inevitable? They were all questions I didn't have answers to.

When we met, the genetics counselor showed me how information I'd sent in about my family history of cancer had been mapped onto a family tree. Instances of cancer were highlighted, but in my case there weren't many. In fact, only one relative on my mother's side of the family had cancer, and none on my father's side. Because of that lack of family history, the counselor said she thought there was only a 5 percent chance of testing positive as a carrier for the BRCA1 or BRCA2 gene. "Regardless, we'll go ahead with the test," she said.

I realized I would be well into chemotherapy before I'd find out the results. Before I left JCC that day, I had to have more blood drawn. I was rapidly becoming oblivious to all the poking and prodding that was being done to my body. Although needles pinched on occasion, of course, I simply endured them, watching as if what was going on was happening to someone else. I couldn't help but stare, however, as the vial filled up with my blood. It seemed as though my entire future rested on that small tube.

On Friday, November 12, Greg and I went to meet with my oncologist, Doctor 7. I felt more prepared for this appointment than any other I'd had, since I already knew I'd likely need chemotherapy. I also had a list of questions in hand, thanks to a wonderful program called CAREpath that I'd enrolled in through my long-term disability benefits. I wasn't yet receiving disability benefits, as I was on maternity leave, but would be when that ended in February on Rudy's first birthday.

The program was optional, but I'd already figured out that second (and third) opinions were never a bad thing, and it meant I could talk to an oncology nurse over the phone about any or all of my treatment options. Shortly after calling for the first time, I was hooked up with a nurse named Margo. She was incredibly knowledgeable and compassionate, which was absolutely what I needed, and talking to her made me feel more comfortable about everything that was happening to me. She also e-mailed me that list of questions. They were great, because I never knew what to expect or ask, and the questions were ones I would never have even thought of myself.

The other great thing about Margo was that I felt like I didn't have to be strong with her. I could let my guard down and expose my fears and frustrations. I didn't want to cry in front of anyone else, for fear that it would show me as being weak, but I cried to Margo on the phone. She wasn't a rookie. She understood.

I soon learned that oncology visits are all about routine. When we arrived at the oncologist's office, we met with a nurse, who checked my weight. As I stood on the scale, I thought about a woman we'd seen in the waiting room, who was clearly going through chemotherapy, had obviously lost a great deal of weight, and looked extremely weak. Right then I made a decision that I wouldn't allow myself to lose any weight during the course of my treatments.

"How much do I weigh?" I asked. I was wearing boots, and even made a point of having the nurse document that in my chart, so that when they compared my weight from one week to the next, the numbers wouldn't be skewed.

Afterwards, a second nurse gave us a detailed overview of what the doctor would say. Greg and I thought that was odd at first, but realized that the practice of meeting with the nurse, then the doctor, ensured nothing would be missed. It also saved time: the nurse could present the doctor with the rundown of the situation as well as any questions we had before we even came face-to-face. Each visit would be the same: weigh-in, questions with a nurse, then the visit with the doctor. The nurse then began running through my chemotherapy schedule. "Drugs are normally administered six times, three weeks apart," she said, "but because of your age and because we want to be aggressive with your treatment, you'll receive what we call dose-dense chemotherapy—eight sessions, two weeks apart."

Yes, let's be aggressive! I thought.

She said that my drug regimen would most likely be a combination called ACT—the first four treatments would be a blend of Adriamycin/doxorubicin and cyclophosphamide and that the last four would be Taxol—and began to list the potential side effects. There were a lot: the expected hair thinning and loss, a decrease in the count of red and white blood cells and platelets, decreased appetite, mouth sores, taste changes, muscle aches, bone pain, severe sunburn with sun exposure, changes in menstrual cycle, including possible early-onset menopause, bladder irritation, allergic reactions, numbness and/or tingling in fingers and toes, diarrhea, discolored urine, nail changes and nasal congestion, among others. But, she cautioned, "Everyone reacts differently. Not everyone experiences all the side effects. Some people don't experience any of them."

I crossed my fingers, hoping I was the latter. But I was worried. The side effects sounded daunting. There was so much to take in. And I thought I'd been so prepared for this appointment!

"If you ever have a fever," the nurse said, "you need to go directly to the emergency room. That's the most important thing to remember."

Greg caught my eye. If she sounded serious before, now she really sounded serious.

"A fever means there's an infection in your body that you can't fight, and only intravenous antibiotics will be able to get rid of it."

By the time Doctor 7 arrived, we felt inundated, and we still had a tour of the chemo suite to come. She was beautiful: long dark hair tied back in a ponytail, glowing skin, nicely dressed. She didn't spend much time getting acquainted. She talked briefly about the chemo schedule, confirmed that I would be on the dose-dense ACT regimen the nurse had mentioned, as long as my white blood cell count stayed up and I stayed healthy, then asked if I had any questions.

"No questions," I said. I think I was in denial.

"When would you like to start?"

"Today." I shifted so I was literally sitting on the edge of my seat.

She smiled. "I can have you start on Tuesday."

Tuesday, meaning the next Tuesday, meaning only four days away. I turned to Greg. The sooner it began, the sooner it would be finished. There was no turning back. Finishing was all I cared about.

Chapter 11

WELCOME TO CHEMO!

∽

*T*he pre-chemo *waiting* room was not at all what I expected. I had imagined a somber, dim room filled with silent, sad people. The opposite was true. It was like a party, with music playing, nurses laughing, volunteers handing out coffee and cookies, visitors knitting, the sun shining through big floor-to-ceiling windows, and so many people.

It was incredibly frustrating to grasp how many people were suffering through the same adversity. And although I was definitely one of the younger people in the room, I wasn't the youngest. "What are we doing wrong?" I asked Greg as we hesitated in the doorway. "Why is this happening to all of us?" Of course he didn't have answers, any more than I did.

A woman came up to us. "Hi, I'm Margaret, a volunteer for the Canadian

Cancer Society," she said warmly. She looked to be in her eighties. "You're new—you get a quilt! Everyone gets one as a welcome gift. While people are waiting, they knit squares." She waved at the baskets scattered here and there about the room, filled with balls of yarn and finished squares. "Then all of the squares are joined together in quilts."

While I chose a quilt, Margaret tossed in what I discovered was one of her signature dirty jokes

"What did the egg say to the boiling water?"

I couldn't begin to guess.

"'Don't expect me to get hard. I just got laid this morning.'" She laughed a wonderful laugh and everyone around us smiled.

This place, which had the potential to be incredibly depressing, was just the opposite. I was so relieved. I would be spending a lot of time here in the upcoming months.

Greg and I took a number and sat in the reception area, waiting to be called to discuss the following Tuesday's treatment.

"It seems odd they call you by numbers instead of names, doesn't it?"

"I know. I wonder why?"

"I guess if you think about it, not everyone wants other people to know they have cancer. There's a stigma attached to illness of any kind, but especially that."

"Although if you didn't have cancer, you definitely wouldn't be called. We know why everybody's here."

"But not their names," I pointed out.

"True."

It was good to have a chance to relax. We had left the oncologist's office feeling optimistic, if saturated with information. Everything had happened so fast that I'd already been given prescriptions for drugs I'd need to take in combination with my chemotherapy treatments. There were four: dexamethasone, an anti-inflammatory steroid used mainly to decrease allergic reactions but also to prevent nausea; Kytril, also to prevent nausea; Neulasta, a needle that would be injected into my stomach three days after treatments to boost white blood cells to prevent infection; and Zopiclone, a sleeping pill that Margo from CAREpath suggested I get to counteract the effects of the steroids I'd be on.

We were lucky everything was so close together—the oncologist's office, the pharmacy and the chemo suite were all on the same floor of JCC and right around the corner from each other—so we'd gone by the pharmacy on the way to the chemo suite to drop off my prescriptions. "They'll be ready by the time you're back," the pharmacist had kindly said.

I couldn't imagine how tiring it would be to spend time driving from place to place all around the city. Greg was already spending huge amounts of time away from work, and so was my mother. I thought about her. She was home with the kids. I knew she felt helpless, that it was difficult for her not to be with me, to be sitting at home instead, waiting, wondering, worrying.

The kids weren't worried. They were too young to know or understand what was going on, and in many ways, because of that, they kept me looking forward, and kept everyone busy, which was a blessing. I'd been run off my feet with the usual chores the last four days trying to get everything organized—I had that list of side effects in mind—because who knew how I'd be feeling after this?

> The kids weren't worried. They were too young to know or understand what was going on, and in many ways, because of that, they kept me looking forward . . . which was a blessing.

I sighed. *Being sick takes a lot of time and effort*, I thought.

⁂

Greg had grabbed a muffin and juice from one of the carts the volunteers were pushing around. He was starving, as usual. He wasn't skinny because he didn't eat, he just had a high metabolism. In fact, when he grabbed the muffin, it reminded me of when I was in labor with Charley. Greg was so hungry, he couldn't help but wolf down a sandwich just moments after Charley was born.

I was shaking my head at the memory when my number was called. I went up to the reception desk, and the woman standing there introduced herself as Anne Marie. She asked me to verify my name and birthdate, then asked if I wanted a tour.

"Absolutely, but is it okay if I bring my husband?"

"Your husband? Which one is he?"

I pointed Greg out.

Anne Marie walked over to where Greg was waiting. Although she'd obviously never met him before, she said, "Are we going to have to put up with you eating all the time? Is this what you're going to be doing every time you come here? Put your food down and come with me!"

I couldn't help but laugh out loud. Maybe that's why I immediately took a liking to Anne Marie. I loved her sarcasm, and the fact that she could joke around with people to lighten the mood. Right away she nicknamed me, which I thought was great.

She showed us the two rooms where people received treatments and explained that I would either sit in a chair (a comfortable-looking recliner) or lie on a stretcher, depending on my treatment. Each room had about twenty-five spaces for patients. Every chair or stretcher was full or being prepped for the next patient. Some patients had someone else sitting with them for company, and some were alone, which I found upsetting. As we walked about, it occurred to me that everyone was looking at us. I wondered why. Could they tell I had cancer? Was it my age? I swiftly realized it was the quilt. Everyone could spot newcomers because of their quilts.

"The Taxol treatments take up to five hours, and having food is essential," Anne Marie said, so she showed us a mini kitchen area where we could keep or warm up food, and a fridge that was stocked full of juice and snacks for patients. She also showed us the bathrooms, and a room where warm towels were kept.

"What are those for?" I asked.

"We use them as blankets, but also to wrap around patients' arms before we start IVs," Anne Marie said. "It gets the veins nice and juicy."

One thing was certain—I was learning a lot.

After our tour we went back to the pharmacy. I was in for a shock when I looked at the receipt for the prescriptions. I nudged Greg and showed him. Every Neulasta injection cost approximately $2,500, and the other drugs weren't cheap, either, though they weren't as incredibly expensive. I needed eight injections in total of the Neulasta and did a quick calculation.

"That's $20,000 right there," I said in disbelief. It had never occurred to me to find out how much the drugs would cost.

"We're lucky your drug plan will cover it."

The pharmacist overheard us and explained that there was an alternative version that the provincial health care plan would cover completely. The difference was that it meant a total of sixty-four needles instead of just eight. I breathed a sigh of relief. But I worried for those who weren't covered.

When we walked out of the pharmacy, me clutching the bag with those valuable drugs, a woman passing by said, "Keep your head up, girl."

At first I wondered if I knew her. Then I realized that once again the quilt had given me away. I hesitated, but I had to know. "Excuse me," I asked. "Are you undergoing chemotherapy, too?"

"I started two weeks ago," she said.

We chatted some more, and she added that she felt fine and hadn't had any side effects, which was reassuring. I couldn't stop thinking about her after we left. She was so upbeat about the whole experience. She didn't have to say anything to me, so why had she? Perhaps she saw something in me that reminded her of herself? When she left, she told me to stay positive. Maybe she knew that in order for me to get through this, I would have to focus all my energy on doing just that.

Doubts gnawed away at me, though. There were only four days until my treatment began. Could I do this?

Chapter 12

THE RED DEVIL

℘

Tuesday morning arrived too quickly.

"I don't know if I'm ready," I said to Greg.

"You can do this," he replied.

Greg was a good person to have around in these kinds of circumstances. He was okay seeing blood or any kind of medical procedure. After all, he'd been a volunteer in the fire department and had done a year in college training as a paramedic. But I wasn't sure about myself. "It reminds me of when I went to the hospital to deliver Rudy," I said as we got in the car. I didn't know how to explain it better than that. Rudy had been eleven days late. I had to go to the hospital to be induced, but I felt perfectly fine. Within a few short hours of being admitted, though, I was in an excruciating amount of pain. What if this was similar? Yet I also felt weirdly upbeat—I was ready to face whatever was coming. I fiddled with the radio, then to keep busy texted some friends.

When we arrived at JCC, a nurse weighed me. "From here, you'll get blood work done, then meet your oncologist before your chemo. That will happen every time you come in."

I made a note in my notebook. I remembered we'd been told about the routine during my first visit, but it couldn't hurt to jot it down. I'd started noting down even more things: questions I had for doctors, nurses, technicians; the numbers regarding my weight and various blood counts; even the amounts we were paying for parking and gas. We'd started saving money before my maternity leave because we knew my paychecks would be cut, but that was before my diagnosis, and things were getting tighter than anticipated because of all the unexpected expenses. I tucked the notebook away. Someone usually accompanied me to appointments, and I often got that person to take notes, since many times I was too emotional to catch everything.

The blood work took only five minutes once we got to the lab.

"You won't always be in and out this quickly," the nurse warned. "There are a lot of people waiting some days."

"How long can it take?"

"Up to thirty minutes, especially if you're here first thing in the morning."

"I'll have to warn whoever's coming with me that they'll definitely have to take the whole day off from work," I said to Greg while we walked down the hallway. I wondered if that would make people change their minds. It was a big commitment.

At the oncologist's office, a woman named Leslie greeted us. "I'm the head nurse. I'll be here most days when you're in, so I'm sure you'll get tired of seeing me."

Like everyone else, she was so friendly. Greg and I followed her to the exam room, and I whispered to him along the way, "I'm so glad I'll have the same nurse—she'll get to know me and how I'm doing." I also liked the fact that she was just wearing a lab coat over regular clothes, as did most of the other doctors and nurses at JCC. This seemed less clinical than scrubs.

We made ourselves comfortable; then Leslie asked, "Have you brought along your nausea pills?"

I showed her my bag. "I think of it as my treasure trove—they're so expensive."

She laughed. "Don't take them yet, because we don't know exactly what time your IV will be. Once they call you into the chemo suite, the nurse there will give you the okay."

"I definitely have to take them?"

"It's best to wait just in case."

Leslie ran through all of the possible side effects that could occur between treatments, including nausea, fatigue and weight loss. "Most are cumulative and could be worse next time. If any occur and become bad, we can certainly tweak your pre-meds next time to help. Most important, if you get a fever at all, you must get to the hospital right away." She paused, letting the information sink in, then asked, "Do you have any questions?"

We'd heard everything before, and could only wait to see what happened. I shook my head.

Doctor 7, my oncologist, came in just as Leslie got up to leave. She was as nice as I remembered, but businesslike. "I know Leslie has already gone over most of this. We'll monitor your blood counts, specifically red and white blood cells, hemoglobin and leukocytes. There's a certain range all of those should stay within."

I asked what the ranges were and made close notes. If I kept track of all the numbers, I thought, maybe I'll be in control. "Logically, I know that doesn't make sense," I said to Greg as we left and walked to the chemo suite. "But emotionally, it makes me feel so much better."

When we checked in at the chemo reception, I was asked if I was going ahead with the treatment. "Sorry?" I said, entirely taken aback.

"We ask that because the drugs aren't mixed until you arrive and check in," the receptionist said. "Even then, it takes a while for them to be ready."

"Oh." That made sense. "Yes, I'm definitely going ahead." I signed the form she gave me. "How long will I have to wait?"

"Depends. Usually a half an hour, sometimes an hour if there are a lot of patients." She handed me my number.

Greg and I sat and waited. We waited forever. I was sure I was the youngest person there. I leaned against Greg and he put his arm around me. Most of the women wore scarves to cover their heads. Their skin looked pale, and it was clear they were well into treatment. When would I become pale? What would I look like without hair? I wondered how many of the people waiting their turn would survive. The room was quiet, so Greg and I stopped talking and simply watched as patient after patient was called in for their turn.

After about an hour and fifteen minutes, my number was called. Greg and I stood up. I took hold of his hand. The nurse who called my number led us into the chemo suite and showed me to a lounge chair. Right away, another nurse came over and handed me a paper cup. "Here's some juice for you to take your pre-meds with," she said.

I took out my medicine bag and counted out the pills—five dexamethasones and one Kytril. I swallowed them all.

Greg watched me. "I don't know how you can take so many at a time."

"If I took them one at a time, I'd need another glass of juice to get them all down."

I noticed the nurse had a towel, and I recalled what our tour guide, Anne Marie, had said about juicy veins during our first visit. "Could you use my right side for the IV?" I asked. "I had lymph nodes removed from my left arm." I knew anything on my left arm, such as a needle or a blood pressure cuff, could increase the chances of lymphedema, or fluid retention.

"Of course," she said, and expertly wrapped my arm.

The towel was nice and warm. "That feels great," I said.

"It really helps."

"What do you do if you can't get good veins?"

"We have to put in something called a PICC line or port catheter."

"What are those?"

"They're placed in either the upper part of your chest or arm so an IV can be directly inserted into the port, not through your skin. But they can't get wet, so showering is an issue, and you have to have a nurse flush them out every so often."

"Not sure I'd want that," I said.

I watched her as she injected the IV needle. I had to—always felt it essential to watch when it came to needles. Perhaps because I was afraid I'd jump if I felt it and hadn't seen it coming.

"In about a half an hour, we'll start the chemotherapy drugs," the nurse said and left.

With Greg's help, I got the lounger reclined all the way back. "It's so comfortable," I said. "I could fall asleep." And I could have if I hadn't been somewhere where everyone was getting cancer treatments. Where I was going to be getting cancer drugs shortly. It was so strange. But the nurses were wonderful, stopping by and offering me a pillow and a blanket and asking if there was anything else I needed.

"Do I look nervous?" I asked Greg.

"You don't," he said with a smile.

He had so much confidence in me. I could feel it. I shut my eyes. Then heard a voice.

"Hi there, I'm Jane. I'm going to get you going on what we call the AC cocktail."

"Cocktail—that's a rather ironic name," I said.

"It is, isn't it?" she said. She turned to Greg. "Would you mind getting some ice chips from the machine around the corner?"

"Sure."

"They help prevent mouth sores by keeping the blood vessels in your mouth from being affected by the medicine."

I pulled out my notebook and hurriedly scrawled down what she'd said. Jane saw what I was doing and had more suggestions. "Change toothbrushes every week during the course of the chemotherapy, too. Rinse your mouth frequently with salt water or baking soda in the days following chemo, and drink lots of water right after the treatment to get the medicine out of your system."

Greg brought back the ice chips, and I started sucking on them.

"First up is the A part of things, or Adriamycin." Jane held up a giant syringe filled with bright red liquid. "Also known as Red Devil."

"That sounds scary," I said.

"It's called that because it's hard on your veins. Normally, with most chemo drugs we just hook up the IV and come back to check on you every once in a while. But with this, we have to push it from the syringe into the IV or port, because it can cause the IV to pop out."

That frightened me. I was glad Greg was sitting beside me, holding my hand. "How long have you worked here?" I asked Jane as she began pushing the drug through the syringe. I was desperate to think of anything other than the drug hitting my body.

"I've been at this hospital for three years, but I worked in the chemo suite at Princess Margaret Cancer Centre before that for eight years."

"How do most people react to AC?" I was babbling but couldn't stop.

"Everyone reacts differently. It's hard to predict."

She was so nice to humor me. I think she realized how I was feeling. I'm sure I wasn't the first person to be frightened.

"Are you feeling all right?"

"So far so good." I'd expected the drug to burn or hurt somehow as Jane started injecting it, so I was happy to be able to say that. I was anxiously thinking about the side effects, though: When would they come and what would they be?

Twenty minutes later, the syringe was empty.

"That was okay, wasn't it?" Jane asked.

I nodded, took a deep breath. The C part of the cocktail, or cyclophosphamide, was still to come. It was in a bag. Jane hung that from a metal stand and connected the tube to my IV. "Oh my god, what is that feeling?" I asked, though, when the infusion started.

"What feeling? What's wrong?" Jane asked.

"My sinuses. They feel weird." I had the strangest sensation, similar to when you get water up your nose while swimming.

"Oh, that. That's normal. It's nothing to worry about," she said. "I'll be back to check on you in a little bit."

"It's such an odd feeling," I said to Greg once she was gone. "I can't shake it." To distract myself, I checked out the people around me. They ranged in age from early twenties to at least eighty years old. Men and women alike. Cancer clearly didn't discriminate. Many patients were sleeping. Some had company, but again, I saw some who didn't. How could anyone send a loved one for treatment alone? The nurses often walked past and smiled, asking if everything was okay. I said yes, but that wasn't true. I thought, *This isn't fair. It isn't okay that I'm here. That any of us is here.* But what could I do? What could any of us do?

Before I'd thought possible, the IV bag was empty and Jane was back. When she removed the IV needle, she asked me to apply pressure to the spot where it had been. "Just for a minute to prevent bruising."

I did so, then got up and began to walk around. Right away, my sinuses began to clear. "How bizarre," I said to Greg. "I feel absolutely fine now." I was thrilled. We still had another stop—the pharmacy to pick up my prescriptions for the next round of chemo—but all in all, the whole treatment took less than an hour. "I can't wait to sit down and cuddle the kids," I told Greg as we made our way out.

"How are you feeling?" He asked as we waited to pay for the drugs.

"Like my body has been pumped full of super toxic drugs—which it has. I just want to do what the nurses said and start drinking lots of water, and then rest." It was almost three P.M., and we'd been gone since eight A.M. It had already been an incredibly long day, and it wasn't over yet.

Mom was at the door when we got home, but I rushed past her. "Sorry, I have to go to the bathroom really badly." I'd drunk at least three bottles of water in the car and the Red Devil was taking effect—the urine in the toilet was tinted red. I'd been told to expect that, but it was weird to see. I flushed, then flushed again, as instructed, to clear the toxic waste from our plumbing system. I shuddered. If the drugs I'd been given could make our house unsafe, what were they doing to my body? I put on a smile, though, as I made my way out to the family room. There was no sense stressing anyone else out.

"How did everything go?" Mom was waiting for me, full of questions.

"Great. I'm just a little tired," I said. "Where are the kids?" I wanted to talk about something other than myself.

"Napping."

That was a relief. I was too tired to play with them.

"Dinner's going to be here in a minute," Greg said. "Gabby's on her way."

"Dinner?" Mom asked.

"You remember I told you about the Dinner Club?" I said. "That group of friends who are going to bring us dinner every other night? It was my friend Kelly's idea, and she and her husband, Andrew, had organized the whole thing. Tonight is Gabby's turn." Seven couples in total were teaming up to deliver our family dinners over the course of the chemotherapy sessions.

"That's so generous," Mom said.

"I know. I can't believe it." I walked to the basement door. "Before Gabby shows up, I'm just going to send a quick e-mail to some family and friends." I needed some time alone. I escaped downstairs, turned on my computer and began typing.

Hello, everyone,

I just got home from my very first chemo session and wanted to let you know how it went. I feel good—a little stoned, maybe, but great!

It's interesting, sitting in a room with everyone in the same situation. Makes you realize you're not alone—and that there are people who have a lot more to complain about than you. I guess that's where my positive attitude comes from—everything could be much, much worse!

I'll keep you posted as much as I can, but that's all for now. I'm going to catch up on a little Oprah—until the kids wake up, of course!

Talk to you later!

As I'd been typing, I began to feel a little nauseous. Correction: I began to feel incredibly nauseous. I rushed to the bathroom and vomited. A lot. I thought I was never going to stop. Finally I did. I hunched over the sink, trembling, and cleaned myself up. I knew Gabby must have arrived and everyone would wonder where I was, so I climbed up the stairs, clutching the rail the whole way.

"Hey, Gabby!" Once again I plastered a smile on my face.

"Alana! You look great!" She gave me a hug. "How did it go? You seem to be doing well."

"Thanks, Gabby." I tried to sound enthused. She was always so kind, I didn't know if she was being thoughtful or if she truly couldn't see what I'd been through. "What did you bring?"

"Orzo pasta with grilled veggies and fresh Parmesan cheese. And a salad for you with some of my homemade dressing."

"That sounds amazing. I hope you didn't go to too much trouble."

"No, not at all! I was making dinner anyway, so I just doubled it."

Charley ran in and grabbed me. "You hungry, sweetie?" I asked after I kissed her. I wasn't sure I was up for eating anything, but I tried to hide it as best I could. "Gabby cooked us dinner and is staying to eat with us!" She nodded and smiled.

Mom chimed in. "Rudy's getting hungry, too, Alana." He was wriggling in her arms.

"Let's have dinner, then." We set the table and chatted as we worked, and by the time we sat down, I felt somewhat better. I was happy, and I was famished. Gabby is Italian, and anything she cooks is delicious. Her orzo dish smelled delicious, and I wanted to eat it. I took a few nibbles and listened while Mom, Gabby and Greg got caught up. Suddenly I put the fork down.

"Would you excuse me?" I could barely get the words out as I pushed back my chair, and everyone stared at me in surprise. I barely made it to the bathroom and vomited again. When I felt better, I emerged. Everyone had abandoned the dinner table, and Gabby was heading to the door.

"I'm so sorry, Gabby," I said. I felt awful, as though I'd ruined the party. "The pasta was so delicious. I'm just not feeling that well."

"Don't worry, Alana. It's not your fault." She gave me another big hug.

I leaned against the door after she left and smiled wanly at Mom and Greg.

"You okay?" Mom asked.

"I just need to rest a bit." I sat on the couch.

The kids followed me, but my mother said, "Charley, play with Rudy and let Mommy sleep," and she and Greg cleaned up.

I managed to relax, but an hour later, as I was trying to get the kids ready for bed, I ran to the master bathroom and vomited again. Shortly after I got there, I heard a knock on the door. It was my mother. I was so sick I couldn't respond. She opened the door and slipped inside.

"I can't stop throwing up," I managed to say.

She pulled my hair back and held it for me. "Maybe you should take more of those pills they gave you for nausea."

"No, I'm sure it'll pass. I'll be fine." It did pass, but I felt so shaky, I went to lie down again. When I felt a bit better, I called Gabby.

"Thank you so much for the amazing dinner," I said. "It's wonderful having food here for everyone so we don't have to worry about that. And I wanted to apologize. I'm sorry I wasn't better company."

"Honestly, don't worry about it. You'll eat when you feel better, and if not, I'll make it for you again sometime. I'm so happy to help."

Although she dismissed it as no big deal, it was a huge deal to me. "Thank you" was all I could manage to say before hanging up and running for the bathroom again. This time in the midst of it, Greg came in to check on me.

"It's okay," I insisted. "Go to bed. I'll be all right." He had to work the next morning and there was no point in both of us being up late. So he did and fell asleep. But I couldn't stop vomiting. I threw up every forty-five minutes, then every half hour. I was in denial, believing it would stop on its own. But by two A.M., I was vomiting every ten minutes.

My mother came upstairs and tiptoed into our bathroom. I was curled around the toilet. I could only glance at her briefly before I began throwing up again, barely able to hold my head up.

"Alana, this is crazy," she said. She'd been downstairs in the spare room, which was right underneath our bedroom, and could hear everything. "I don't care what you say. We're going to the hospital."

Chapter 13

DO THEY STAY OR
DO THEY GO?

*M*om practically dragged me to the car. The drive was a blur. Once we got to the hospital, she took charge, and I was admitted quickly. The emergency room was so bright. I just wanted to curl up and die. I heard voices somewhere beside me.

"Get her on saline and an antinauseant."

I groaned as they hooked me up to yet another IV. I could hear Mom talking.

"How long will it take to work? She's been throwing up almost constantly."

"Pretty fast. Once we get her rehydrated, she'll start feeling better. We'll give her something to help her sleep, too."

I was aware that Mom sat down beside me and took my hand. Then whatever they gave me must have started working. I slept until morning, Mom took me home, and I crawled right back into bed. When I woke up later that morning, Mom brought me something to eat.

"It's just dry toast. I don't want you to start vomiting again," she said as she set the tray down.

"What did they give me last night? I feel better, I think," I said as I cautiously started nibbling the toast.

"Something called Zofran. I asked them about it and they said it's an extremely effective yet very expensive antinauseant," she said, watching me carefully. "Most doctors know it works well, but they don't usually prescribe it because of the cost. And they don't know immediately if every patient will need it." She fluffed up a pillow and sat down beside me. "They also gave you some Ativan to help you relax and sleep."

"Whatever the combination was, it worked. Thankfully." I drank some water and started on another slice of toast. Mom raised an eyebrow.

"So far, so good," I said. "Apparently I have expensive taste."

She smiled.

We were overly optimistic. The vomiting started up again and continued on and off for another forty-eight hours, but it wasn't anywhere near as bad or frequent as it had been the night before. Greg and Mom kept bringing me food, though. They both knew I was determined to maintain my weight, and the whole bout of vomiting had thrown that off. By about the third day after chemo, the nausea started to go away enough that I could begin to eat normally again. And just in time: that day I had to get my Neulasta injection, the first of eight I would need. While the chemotherapy would help rid my body of cancer, it could also lower my white blood cell count. Neulasta would force my bone marrow to produce more of those cells. My mother would be giving me the injections, but a nurse was coming by to demonstrate the procedure to her.

"Here she is!"

The nurse was friendly but efficient, and began unpacking her supplies the minute she came in. "What time of day are you planning to do the injection?" she asked.

"In the afternoon, when my son is down for a nap, so there won't be any distractions."

"Any other time would be impossible," Mom added.

"It's true. The kids would be either running around or trying to grab the needle while Mom's injecting it!"

"Whenever you decide to do it," the nurse said, "just remember to always take the syringe out of the fridge approximately a half hour before you're ready." She took the syringe off the kitchen counter. Mom had taken it out of the refrigerator prior to her arrival, as instructed. "It's prefilled. With one hand, squeeze the skin on her tummy into a fold like this." She grabbed my stomach and showed my mother, who leaned over me to watch. "Using the other hand, firmly jab the needle into the skin, then push the plunger." With that, she injected me.

"You think you can do that?" I asked my mother.

"Looks straightforward to me."

I wasn't sure she sounded convinced, but she knew she needed to be able to do this, and she was determined.

"Just to clarify, the needle is ready to go? All I have to do is push the plunger to make it go into her skin?"

"You got it. Alana, you might feel a bit sore in the injection site for a day or two after, and there might be a bit of bruising, but it shouldn't be too bad." She looked at my mother. "Just remember where you injected and use a different spot each time."

"Is there anything else we should know?" I asked.

"The drug may make your bones ache somewhat, but you should be fine otherwise."

Neither of us had any other questions, so the nurse went on her way, giving me a hotline number we could call if we had any problems. I shut the door after her. "Are you sure you're okay with the idea of giving me the needle, Mom?"

"Of course. I just hope you feel all right after," she said distractedly. I could tell she was worried that she'd do something that would cause me discomfort on top of everything else.

Charley, on the other hand, was oblivious to how I was feeling much of the time.

"Mom, can we go to the park?" she asked one sunny but cold afternoon when I was lying on the couch.

"Charley, I'll take you and Rudy when he wakes up from his nap," my mother jumped in. "Let Mommy rest."

"I'll go, too," I said. I was tired. I would have liked to rest. I probably should have rested. But how could I say no to my child? How on earth would Charley understand it if I kept saying no? What if cancer ultimately took my life? How would she remember me? As the mother who always said no? So off we went after getting the kids dressed and tucking Rudy in his stroller.

"One more time, Mommy!" Charley yelled as she got to the bottom of the slide for the umpteenth time. When she ran back around to the ladder again, she said, "Come with me!"

"Who me?" I hesitated for no more than a split second before I climbed up with her. We played until even the kids got tired, then headed home. "That truly was just what I needed," I said to my mother. As we walked, I couldn't help but think about what had already occurred, and what was looming over me. The fate of my breasts.

"Mom," I said, breaking my silence, "if you knew that keeping your breasts increased your risk of having cancer, what would you do?"

> How could I say no to my child? How on earth would Charley understand it if I kept saying no? What if cancer ultimately took my life? How would she remember me? As the mother who always said no?

She stopped walking and took me by the arms. "Alana, you need to do whatever it is that you need to do. If it means removing your breasts, then remove your breasts. If you need to remove a finger or a toe as well, do it. I want you here for a long time and so do your kids."

I hadn't realized it, but I'd been holding my breath. I released it in a big cloud of white smoke that drifted off into the winter sky. "You're right. I was thinking the same thing. I just didn't know if that was too drastic."

"Not at all. And if it was me, I would tell the doctors to take both."

I hadn't had an in-depth discussion with my doctors about a mastectomy, but the decision turned out to be not so difficult after all. I felt relieved. We'd been out playing for more than an hour, and the time had flown by. I was tired but glad I'd gone. There was no question in my mind anymore. The situation was desperate, and I would resort to desperate measures because I had to.

That night at dinner I said to Greg and my mom, "I'm going to ask for a double mastectomy. I don't want these anymore, and I don't want to be at any kind of elevated risk." I waited for them to interject, but somehow I knew they wouldn't. They knew me well enough to know that once I had made up my mind, there wasn't going to be any convincing me otherwise.

Chapter 14

IT'S ONLY HAIR, ISN'T IT?

⤳

*W*hen *I was* growing up, there were plenty of times when I wanted to be like everyone else, especially during those formative teenage years. I wanted to wear what everyone else was wearing, I wanted to look like everyone else, and I especially wanted the same brand-name items everyone else had—from clothes to purses to shoes.

My mother held another point of view. "You should appreciate being different from other people, being unique in some way," she'd say. Erin, Braden, and I didn't always have a choice—Mom did the majority of the shopping for us.

As an adult, I was determined to put what Mom tried to teach us into practice. That meant trying not to feel down about eventually losing my hair, but rather embracing that situation. "I'm thinking about having a head-shaving party," I said to my good friend Michael, who was also my chiropractor. When the time came for my hair to go, I wanted be the one to get rid of it. I didn't want to leave that to the cancer or the chemotherapy. "That way my friends and family can be there with me as I cut it all off. What do you think?"

"When you do it, I'll do it, too," he said.

"Really? Come on." I was half laughing to myself at the thought of him being bald, yet was almost positive he was joking.

"Absolutely. I'm 100 percent in. We'll do it together."

A few days later, my friend Andre stopped by my house after he was done teaching. He'd been my teaching partner for five years and we were close. Even though I was off on maternity leave, we kept in touch, talking and often getting together. "I heard what Michael's going to do," he said. The two of them were good friends, too.

"Crazy, isn't it?"

"Not at all! I'm going to help him plan the party."

"What?"

"We're totally with you, Alana."

I hugged him. My crazy friends!

Michael and Andre rallied even more of my friends, including Melanie and a number of the other teachers I worked with, and began organizing everything.

"Tony booked the venue," Andre said. "We're going to have it at Dave & Buster's." Tony was another of my colleagues, whom I'd gotten along with right from the start. He worked part-time as a bartender on weekends in addition to teaching. "It's got food, drinks, even an arcade for the kids, so something for everyone. It's the perfect place.

"We'll sell tickets, and we figure some of the money can go to help you with your extra costs or to hire someone to help you clean, and some can go to a cancer charity. The price will include food and games. And we'll get friends and family to donate prizes for a silent auction." I could tell he was so excited.

"I can't believe what you guys are doing! You're amazing!" I hugged him and almost started crying. I was so excited, too, that for a moment I almost stopped thinking about the fact that I was going to lose my hair.

I didn't have long to figure out a way to explain that I was going to be losing my hair to Charley. I struggled with that. A lot had to do with how I felt about it. I didn't want to look odd; I wanted to maintain my dignity, to look like a lady.

In the end, I just started talking. "Charley, you know that Mommy isn't feeling well, right?"

She looked at me and nodded.

"I have to take some medicine that's going to make me better."

"Is it purple?"

I knew she was thinking of grape-flavored children's medicine she'd taken when she had a cold. "No, not purple. But you know how we'll know the medicine is working?"

She thought for a minute. "How?"

"Because it will make my hair fall out." I kept talking before she could say anything. "And that's a good thing! If my hair didn't fall out, then we wouldn't know that Mommy's getting better."

"Okay," she said, and went off to play.

My mother had come in as I finished talking. "Either this is over her head," I said to her, "or it's not that big a deal."

"I think children take things as they come."

"You're probably right. This is happening too fast. I hope Charley is okay with everything. As for me, I'm scared to get my head shaved by someone I don't know. I've never had a hairdresser I've called my own."

"Don't worry. I've already taken care of it."

"What do you mean?"

"I've asked Lepa to come to the party."

"That's perfect!" Lepa was Mom's hairdresser. She'd never cut my hair, but I knew her well. Mom thought of everything.

"I'm going to check on the kids," she said. "You take it easy."

I glanced around the room. "I'm not sure that's possible around here." Toys were scattered everywhere as usual. Mom left, and I started cleaning up. I couldn't help but glance in the hall mirror as I passed by it. I pulled my hair back tightly, trying to imagine how I'd look with no hair.

I couldn't.

I couldn't help but glance in the hall mirror as I passed by it. I pulled my hair back tightly, trying to imagine how I'd look with no hair. I couldn't.

❧

I decided to take Charley with me to go look for a wig. The idea of wearing a wig was bizarre. I still had my own hair. On a bulletin board at the JCC I'd noticed a list of wig suppliers, and one was close to my home, so I called to book an appointment. I couldn't wait forever to do this. The man I spoke with, Carlo, was nice. I asked him if I could bring Charley, and he was fine with that, but mysteriously told me to use the side door when I arrived. I wondered why.

I didn't tell Charley where we were going until we were getting ready to leave. "I need your help with something," I said to her as we got dressed. I'd put Rudy down for a nap, and my friend Susanne, who was Greg's boss's wife, had come over to babysit.

"What do you need?"

"Remember when Mommy talked about the medicine? Well, we're going to the wig store so I can buy some fun hair to wear until my own hair grows back. I want you to tell me which looks good."

"Can I try on some, too?"

"Absolutely! As many as you like." I was relieved that she was keen to go.

On the way to the hair salon, Charley had a quick nap and I knew she'd be in even better spirits when she woke up. When we arrived, my mother met us in the parking lot.

"We're supposed to use the side door," I said.

"Why?"

"I don't know." We then discovered that the side door led to a private area attached to the main salon but used only for wig fitting.

"I guess it allows women privacy if they're at all uncomfortable with the process," I said quietly.

Carlo came over. He couldn't have been more welcoming. "You must be Charley," he said as he bent down to greet her.

She was pointing in all directions. "I want to try on that one and that one and that one."

"Thanks for seeing me today, Carlo. I wanted to come last week, but I didn't realize how ill I'd be feeling after that first chemo session."

"You're here now, and we'll find something that's perfect. Please have a seat. Are you planning on sticking with the same style and color you have now?"

Each of the wigs that caught Charley's eye looked drastically different from her own hair. Meanwhile, I hadn't even thought about what I wanted. "I think so."

With that, Carlo got to work. He looked at my hair, felt it, and began taking wigs off the shelves and putting them on my head. Mom kept Charley occupied by pulling down every wig she liked. Trying on wigs was an odd experience. They didn't fit correctly and needed to be stretched and manipulated, and because I still had a full head of hair, they pouffed up at the top. They definitely didn't look like me, that was for sure.

"None of these is going to feel perfect right now," Carlo said. He must have seen the worry on my face. "They'll feel better once your hair is all gone. And I'll cut and style whichever you choose to match your hair now, so it will look much better."

I was surprised. I didn't realize that a wig would be styled to match my look. Even so, they didn't feel like my own hair. As Carlo finished adjusting the tenth wig, I said, "This is the one." The cut wasn't perfect, but the color and texture were as close as I was going to get. Mom took a couple of fun pictures of Charley and me before we left. Was she taking them because she wanted to make sure she had a keepsake for Charley if I didn't make it? I stopped my thoughts mid-track. I wasn't going to go there today. I was going to focus on how glad I was that I had brought Charley along, that we had photos at all. That we'd had a good time. Including Charley in the future whenever possible was the best thing I could do, for her and for me.

♗

I was running out of time. I knew from the experts at JCC that the timing of when a person's hair falls out was quite exact: between seventeen and twenty-one days after chemotherapy begins. I had only a few precious days left to spend with my lovely locks. I needed to decide what to do, to plan how things would go.

"Hey, Lepa, it's Alana. Thank you so much for offering to come to the party to cut my hair. I really appreciate it."

Lepa had been so quick to answer the phone and she almost didn't wait for me to finish talking before she jumped in. "I'm so happy to help. Don't worry at all. I'll give you a nice cut. I don't want to buzz it off. I want to give you a cute haircut. Maybe a pixie cut or something. It will be beautiful."

"Thanks, Lepa. I'm very nervous."

"It will look great. A short haircut will suit you. You have a beautiful face, just like your mom. I'll see you, okay?"

"See you, Lepa. And thank you again." I hung up. Lepa always made my mother's hair look wonderful, so I felt a bit more at ease after speaking with her, but I wasn't excited about any of it. Before I could think about it any more, Charley joined me in the living room. She demanded I stay right where I was. I didn't dare move an inch, even though she left the room.

"Look what I found," she announced as she came back. She had formed a little pouch with her shirt and brought out practically every elastic hairband and barrette that had been in the bathroom drawer.

For the next fifteen minutes, she played with my hair—she'd always loved doing that—twisting and clipping it, and I soaked it all in. When she was done, she sat back and admired her work. "Mommy, you look so pretty!"

We both went to look in the mirror. Bands and barrettes were everywhere, tufts of hair poked out in all directions.

"I do look pretty, Charley, I do." I kissed her. "Thank you. It's beautiful."

She skipped away, and I started crying. Not only was cancer going to take away my hair and my breasts, it was going to take away those special moments—for me and for Charley. The tears kept coming.

Chapter 15

IT'S MY PARTY, AND I'LL CRY IF I WANT TO

$\wp$

My $idea$ of the little head-shaving party for a few friends had ballooned into a bona fide event. Andre and Michael made sure to keep me up-to-date as all their plans fell into place.

"I've arranged for some hairdressers I know to come and work for free," Andre said. "For anyone who wants to join in on the fun of being bald!"

"We've gotten people to donate amazing prizes for the auction—cases of wine, signed NHL hockey sticks, spa treatments, gift certificates and other great things," Michael added.

"I've even worked on setting up a barbershop area in the restaurant for the haircutting."

"And we've sold a ton of tickets," Michael said. "Over two hundred so far!" The two of them were beyond proud. I was so happy for them. They'd done an incredible job and I couldn't wait to see the results. But I couldn't help but feel dismay when November 25, the day of the party, arrived. I had only a few more hours with my long hair. I wanted to head to the bathroom to spend time styling my hair for the last time, but I had Rudy with me and everyone was busy elsewhere.

"You'll ruin all the fun, Rudy," I said as he kept tugging away at my hair, trying to pull it out—and succeeding at times. I was just about to scream when my mother noticed my frustration.

"Here, let me take him."

I gratefully handed Rudy over to her and locked myself in the master bathroom so I wouldn't be disturbed by anyone. I spent more time doing my hair than usual—even separating it into sections when I blow-dried it, the way a hairdresser would. I rubbed a strand between my fingers, trying to absorb how it felt and looked. Somehow it already felt different. There was less of it, for sure. But there was something else I couldn't quite pinpoint—a difference in the texture, perhaps, caused by the chemotherapy? I might just have been imagining it, but whatever it was, I knew it didn't matter. Soon most of it would be gone, anyway.

Only Charley was coming to the party. Since Rudy was only nine months old, we'd decided to leave him at home with a babysitter.

"Hey, Charley, look what Mary Kay sent you!" my mother called out as Charley and I made our way out to the kitchen after getting dressed. "It's a pink ribbon for your hair."

"It matches your outfit, Charley!" I said. She was wearing a dress, as usual. She loved girlie things.

"You look good, Alana," Greg said.

"Thanks." Figuring out what I would wear had been easy. "I can't believe Mary Kay sent me this. She must be psychic."

"What do you mean?" Mom asked.

"A few days ago, I was looking through the T-shirt section at Target and saw this purple T-shirt with the word *Believe* embroidered on it. I loved how sparkly it was, and thought it would be great for the party but decided not to get it since I already had so many T-shirts. Then yesterday a package arrived for me, and it was this!"

"It was a sign," Mom said.

"It was! You know how significant the word *Believe* has become to me with my special project."

Mom nodded.

I had realized early on in this journey how important keeping busy was—it was one of my coping mechanisms. I also knew I didn't like the idea of wearing a scarf around my head to hide any hair loss. I somehow equated this with the idea of being old. But I didn't want to reveal my baldness—I didn't want to look like I had cancer. "I think I'll get fewer looks from people if I wear a toque instead," I'd told my mother one day a few weeks earlier.

"I'll look for one when I'm out. Maybe I'll see something you'll like."

"But I want to have the word *Believe* embroidered on it, with a pink ribbon substituted for the letter *l*." I drew a little sketch of what I was thinking and showed her. "I truly believe cancer isn't going to beat me. I'm going to beat it, and I want the world to know."

"I'm so proud of you, Alana." She surprised me when she started to tear up. "Everyone is going to love that hat."

"They'll all want one."

"They will. You should sell them."

I thought she was kidding, but it dawned on me that she had a great point. "They *will* want one! Andre and Michael are coming up with all those fabulous ways to raise money and offset our costs, so why can't we sell hats to raise money, too? And not everyone who has cancer has the support I do." I thought of the people I'd seen at the chemo suite getting treatment all alone. "Imagine what it's like without a family or friends like ours? We could raise money for a charity like Wellspring, too."

Mom was totally on board, and we got to work. I pulled together a website and showed it to Greg. Wellspring was the perfect charity to give the proceeds to, as it is a network of community-based centers that provide much-needed support to cancer patients and their caregivers.

"Impressive!"

"I want to sell as many *Believe* hats as we can. I can't help but think that the amount of support people get affects how well they cope during treatment. That's why I think I'm handling everything so well—because I have all of you helping me."

The night of the party, I knew the T-shirt was the perfect choice of outfit and would perfectly complement the hats we'd be selling. As we headed out and I shut the door behind me, Mom asked, "You remembered the hats, right?"

"They're already in the car."

"How many do you have?" Greg wanted to know.

"Forty-eight pink ones and forty-eight black."

"Let's hope we sell them all!" Mom said.

"I'm sure we will. I've had so many people tell me they want one."

I was feeling tiny butterflies before we'd even pulled out of the driveway. By the time we arrived at the restaurant, I was downright nervous. My mind was eased only by my previous discussion with Lepa, but my stomach sank at the idea that even a pixie cut would probably fall out within a week or so.

Mom looked at me when we got out of the car.

"I'm a bit tense," I whispered. I didn't want Charley to hear. I ran a hand through my hair. "I hate to admit it, but I realize it's going to feel weird with such short hair."

"You'll always be beautiful, Alana. No matter what," she said, and gave me a quick squeeze before we went into the restaurant.

"Alana!" Andre shouted when he saw me, and he gave me a big hug.

"I love your T-shirt," I said after he let go of me and I could get a good look at what he was wearing. His pink shirt had our school name on it and a picture of a volleyball, but I'd never seen Andre wear pink before. "Where'd you get it?"

"We ordered them for the volleyball teams this year. I know the school colors are blue and white, but we decided to make them pink in honor of you!"

"We?" I looked around. I hadn't noticed because Andre had grabbed me right when I'd walked in, but all the teachers from my school were wearing the pink T-shirts. I could feel myself blushing and waved to everyone. Tony was behind the bar, serving up drinks. "You guys are great." I walked around, saying hi, introducing everyone who didn't know them to my family.

"Alana!"

"Nina!"

Nina and I taught together—I taught eighth grade and Nina sixth—and we were fast friends.

"Don't you love the T-shirts?" she asked.

"They're amazing!"

"Look what I have for you." She handed me a bag.

"You shouldn't have," I said as I took it and opened it. Inside was a T-shirt of my own that read *Boobie Brigade: We Fight Like Girls*.

"I love it, Nina! It's fabulous!"

"Melanie, Virginia, Adriana and I came up with the idea. We talked about it at school and had them made for the five of us."

"You guys are incredible." They had been there for me right from the beginning. They came over one night shortly after my diagnosis and rallied around me, and they had been there for me ever since. I couldn't have made it without them—without their home-cooked meals, their positivity, their support.

"And check this out." Nina waved me over to a table so we could sit down and pulled out her camera. She flicked it on and passed it to me.

"Get well soon, Mrs. Somerville!" I could hear little voices shout. It was the boys' and girls' volleyball teams, all glorious in pink. I choked up.

"Andre had the shirts made in time for me to tape the message," Nina said, then noticed my reaction. "Oh, Alana, I'm so sorry." She wrapped her arms around me.

"No, it's so nice of all of you—and the kids, too. It just seems wrong that kids so young have to hear about cancer. Why should kids that age—or any age—have to deal with that?" I tried to smile. "But this is a party, right?"

"Right!" She put away the camera, and we went to get some drinks from Tony. As we chatted with him, Lepa set up her haircutting station. I sneaked away to talk to her. Andre had done a great job with the "barbershop." There were two barber chairs sitting in front of a roped-off area at the back of the restaurant where everyone would watch the haircuts. I shivered. I would be sitting in one of those chairs soon, facing the crowd, with Lepa standing behind me.

"Lepa, thank you so much for coming," I said and took her hand.

"I am happy to be here, for you and for your mom. How is she?"

"She's keeping it together. She's a rock."

Lepa smiled. "Listen, Alana, when your hair starts growing back in, come see me and I'm going to keep it nice, okay? No charge."

"You're the best. I'm so lucky to have you here." I squeezed her hand.

More people had shown up while I'd been chatting with Lepa, and before I knew it, the restaurant was packed. I mixed, I mingled, I sat for photos. I felt as though I was reliving my wedding: everyone was there for me, everyone wanted to talk to me. Most of them just wanted a chance to connect, and to tell me they were thinking of me. I felt so grateful that people had taken time out of their busy lives.

My friends, some of whom I was seeing for the first time since I'd been diagnosed, were a mixture of curious and cautious. A small group gathered around me. "When is your next round of chemo?" one asked. "How did you feel after surgery?" another inquired. The questions—"What did the lump feel like?" "How did you find it?" "When did you know it was cancer?" and more—flowed from there, the faces growing more and more eager for information as they realized I was happy to respond. In fact, it felt therapeutic. Answering people's questions meant I could do something to help them, letting them know more about this disease.

This was a scene that was repeated many times throughout the evening. The conversations followed the same pattern each time—a movement from generalities to specifics. And almost always the questions came from women. They were interested yet fearful. I figured most of them would go home that night and check their breasts, carefully. I knew they were afraid they'd end up like me. Wanted to reassure themselves they wouldn't.

I understood, but it made me sad. This didn't affect only me anymore. My disease had touched so many people in a way I'd never imagined it would. And for fleeting yet incredibly disturbing moments, I wondered, *Will this be the last time some of my friends and family see me?*

All the while I knew that at some point the haircutting would have to begin. That hovered over me like a horrible creature in a never-ending nightmare. We all talked about anything but the haircut, but everyone knew that's what I was there for, that it was inevitable. Finally the hairdressers were all set up, and the crowd was getting antsy. I wanted to tell someone how scared I was, but I simply couldn't bring myself to say the words out loud.

"Hey." Michael appeared by my side. "Shall we get going?"

I couldn't move. After what seemed like minutes but was surely just a few seconds, he graciously said, "I'll go first." He must have realized how hard the situation was for me. My knees felt like they were going to buckle. He sat down in one of the chairs and Lepa got to work. I couldn't help but stare. It was so odd to watch as his thick beautiful curls fell to the floor. But when it was all over, everyone applauded—he looked great with a buzz cut. He'd handled his haircut with such grace, I realized I could, too, but more people had already kindly lined up ahead of me to give me more time to collect myself. When I sat down, a former student of mine named Brody took a seat in the chair next to me.

"Brody! You're getting your hair done?"

"I am," he said. "I need a haircut."

We both laughed. His hair looked fine, but I knew that was his way of saying he wanted to help me out. What a sweet kid. That was something you couldn't teach in school. And he was so young.

"Are you all set, Alana?" Lepa asked.

"All set!" And I wasn't just saying that. Everyone taking part had given me courage, and everyone I loved—Greg, Charley, and my mother—was right there in the front row with me. "Can you cut a lock for me that I can save?"

"Of course," she said, and she cut a curl and carefully handed it to me.

Then off she went. I could hear the scissors snipping away, feel the hair dropping onto my shoulders, the weight actually falling off my head. All eyes were on me, but I couldn't bring myself to watch. I put on a big smile even though it took a huge amount of effort to keep it in place. I wasn't going to let anyone know how scared I was about how I would look—or what would happen to me in the future.

"You're done," Lepa said, flourishing her scissors. Everyone clapped and said they loved it. I raised my eyes to the mirror.

"I love it, too," I said. But my lips quivered when I saw my reflection. I wanted my long hair back. I clutched the lock in my hand. I didn't want short hair. I didn't want any of this. Lepa had done the best she could—she'd styled what hair was there beautifully—but what I saw in the mirror wasn't me.

"You do look almost like Caillou, Mommy!" Charley said, all excited. She'd been watching TV more often since Rudy was born even though I'd always said I'd never let television be a babysitter for my kids. *Caillou* was the bald-headed main character of a kids' show she watched. "I'm so glad you think so, sweetie." I kissed her.

Greg came up and gave me a hug, then sat down in one of the barber chairs.

"I thought you weren't going to get your hair cut?" I said.

"I changed my mind."

People had asked him, and his answer had always been no. I was so glad to have his support. We were a team. We would do this together. When Lepa was done, Greg looked great. She'd given him a buzz cut! "You look so cute!"

Greg blushed.

"Gloria, you're next!" Lepa said as she motioned for my mom to come sit in the chair.

"I'm ready! Lepa, I want my hair short to match Alana's."

I didn't know she was going to do that. It was the most incredible gesture. "We're going to look like twins!" I said.

The party was turning out to be an evening of surprises. I tucked the lock away in my purse. My uncle Jimmy, my sister-in-law, a teacher I worked with, and a good friend of my mother's all sat down to get a haircut, and after that Brody showed up again.

"What are you doing back here?" Lepa asked him.

"I want my hair cut as short as the clippers can make it."

"That's pretty short."

"Good! That's what I want!"

I turned to my mother as we watched him. "I've realized something tonight. When their hair is gone, it doesn't change who they are. I mean, your hair is so different now, but you haven't changed all of a sudden. You're the same person."

"Of course I am, Alana. And so are you."

"I never knew how much I could learn from someone like Brody. Or Charley. This is turning out to be an experience in ways I never would have imagined." Mom smiled, although I think she also wanted to cry. "I think I might play a little trick on Charley tomorrow morning."

"What kind of trick?"

"Before she wakes up, I'll put a wig on from the Halloween Box with all of the costumes, and tell her that my hair grew back overnight." I was completely joking, but I wanted to keep everyone's spirits up.

Andre's wife, Tina, came by. She'd been handling the hat and raffle ticket sales. She handed me an envelope. "Guess what?" she said. "We sold every single *Believe* hat—all ninety-six!"

"It's amazing! You're amazing," I said. "Everyone here is amazing!"

I glanced at myself in the mirror one last time before we left. My next chemo treatment was the following Tuesday. I had one week to enjoy my new haircut.

Chapter 16

EVERYTHING IS CRAP

$\mathcal{P}$

I had what felt like the biggest support group in the world, the most amazing friends and family who cooked dinners for my family, held hair-cutting parties, helped with errands, and more, and I truly felt blessed. But I often had moments when I found it hard to be positive, when I couldn't help but think how horrible things were.

I didn't like how I looked. I tried to like it. I tried to learn to style my new hair in ways I thought would look good, but it was futile. And I'd started having hot flashes and they were messing with everything, including my sleep. I didn't even realize what they were until my period stopped, which is what clued me in. I never knew when to expect the flashes. I soon figured out that they'd typically start with a chill. I'd get cold, bundle up, then within a minute, I'd be ripping off the sweaters, toque, socks—all of it—because I'd be dripping with sweat. The flashes would last only a couple of minutes, but at night, they made sleep uncomfortable, and whatever sleep I got wasn't a deep, refreshing sleep.

So I felt like crap. I lay low around the house, trying to keep myself busy, and tried not to think about how I felt or about what was to come. Even so, the next week sped by, and I found myself at my second chemo appointment, annoyed because I didn't want time to pass, wanted to hold on to what little I had, even though I hated everything about what was happening.

♏

"You've lost four pounds."

I stared at the nurse in disbelief. I was at the weigh-in, and a vision of the painfully thin woman in the waiting room from my first visit flashed through my head. After all my determination, all I'd said to everyone about not losing weight, there I was.

My oncologist, Doctor 7, wasn't happy, either. "Because you got so nauseated, we'll try you on Zofran," she said.

My mom chimed in. It was her turn on the schedule to accompany me. "That's the drug you got the night I took you to the hospital."

"You'll get it intravenously before the chemo drugs are started," Doctor 7 added, "along with dexamethasone, as before, and Emend, which you'll take orally about an hour before chemo. Then for the next three days you'll take Emend and Zofran orally, along with dexamethasone."

"I guess I have expensive tastes," I joked, desperately trying to see the funny side of things.

"Well, if that doesn't work, we'll even have a home-care nurse come give you antinausea drugs intravenously," she said, playing along.

I wondered if I should ask for a housekeeper while I was at it.

♏

Mom and I picked up the new prescriptions, then headed to the chemo suite. When my number was called, I tried to make myself comfortable as I took the new drugs and the chemo nurse started my IV, but I was having a hard time relaxing. I surreptitiously crossed my fingers as the nurse started pushing the Red Devil through my veins.

"Everything okay?" the nurse asked as she sat there with me, syringe in hand.

"Fine, thanks." As usual, I found sharing my feelings wasn't easy.

"You're nervous," Mom said. She knew I wasn't okay.

"I just hope the new regimen of drugs will do the trick. I definitely don't want to get so violently ill again." She put her hand on my arm and rubbed it. There was nothing either of us could do. We just had to wait and see.

I sat back. There were two young girls sitting on either side of us, and I couldn't help but listen to them as they talked. One was about twenty years old and was there with a guy who said they were dating (she disagreed). They had a slew of board games and were cracking up the whole time. The other girl was quieter, around eighteen years old, and was there with her mother. I whispered to Mom, "I wonder what their stories are."

She shook her head. "Could be anything."

"But we do know they have cancer."

"That, definitely."

The nurse came back to check my vitals.

"How old are the patients you treat here?" I asked quietly.

"Anywhere from sixteen and up. A lot of the young ones are boys with testicular cancer."

I sat for a while when she left again, then looked at my mother. "Whatever rough time I'm going through is nothing compared to what's happening to a lot of people. And when I think about kids that young going through what I am, it's awful." I promised myself I would try to remember that the next time I was feeling down.

❀

"No vomiting—hooray!" I was so happy, I couldn't help cheering to Gabby, who'd come by with another delicious meal. It was three hours after my treatment, and I was feeling fine.

"That's great, Alana. You're making progress every single time. Way to go!"

"The nausea hasn't gone away entirely, but not throwing up is such a welcome change." I was glad, too, because I didn't want to play around with the combination of drugs anymore for fear the vomiting would start up again. "I can handle a bit of nausea. After all, with both of my pregnancies I had constant morning sickness for eight weeks."

"Then you should be able to eat some of this." She dished out some pasta.

"What is it?"

"Chicken Parmesan and rigatoni pasta."

"Gabby, I'm going to gain back all the weight I lost eating just your food."

"Good! That's exactly what I want to hear."

It wasn't even dinnertime yet, but I had to have some. It was delicious. "You have to give me the recipe. When I feel better, I'm going to make this for everyone."

"I'll come over and we'll make it together."

"Deal."

⌒

After Gabby had left and we'd eaten and cleared up, my mother came over to me on the couch to see how I was doing. I was tired, I was definitely nauseous, but at least I wasn't throwing up. She put my feet on her lap and rubbed them the way she did when I was little. "I'm so grateful I'm feeling much better. I can keep food down. I ate such a huge plate of Gabby's food."

"No aches?"

"No, they'll come when you give me my Neulasta needle in a couple of days. But they only last a few days and then I head into my good week.

It seems that exactly one week after treatment, I begin to feel better and get progressively better. That is until the day of the next treatment comes."

"Those needles are payback for me," Mom joked. She'd started telling people she would enjoy giving them to me because I'd given her such a hard time when I was young. I smiled. Like me, she tried to joke about the things in life that were tough, but I knew the truth: She hated the thought of the needles. Hated that she had to hurt me. But she knew each one meant a step closer to the end of chemotherapy.

"You're doing an excellent job taking care of me, Mom. Everyone is."

Even Charley had started "checking up" on me. One night she came into our bedroom, where I was lying down. Although I hadn't outright told Charley that I was feeling sick or complained to her about the side effects of the chemotherapy, she was definitely starting to be more observant, maybe even a little worried.

"How are you, Mommy?"

"Feeling a bit tired tonight, honey. Are you getting ready for bed?" I asked. I kept trying to keep the focus on her, not on me, in our interactions. That was hard if I was feeling particularly ill, but I definitely didn't want her to worry.

"I'm ready. Can you read me a story?" she asked, holding up the book she'd hidden behind her back.

Ever since she was a baby, Greg and I would read to her in her room before bed. Even when she was nursing, I'd tell her stories. It crushed me that I wasn't able to keep up the routine of going into her room, but at the same time I loved that she came to me. Bedtime reading was our time. I knew the location didn't matter. "Of course," I said. No matter how tired I was, how could I say no to that? "Crawl up next to me, and we'll read it together." She did, and I began to feel better. "I wish I could lie here forever with you, Charley."

"Me too, Mommy."

I began to understand why people would want to skip their treatment days, because after all the nausea and horrible feelings start to fade away, you began to feel like yourself again, but you know that the next chemo treatment will make you feel that same horrible way, again and again. I sighed. "It's time for bed, though, honey."

"Now?"

"Yes, now. But we'll read again tomorrow night, I promise."

She got up, tucked me in and gave me a kiss, then picked up her book and left. I watched her walk out. *I would willingly go through the hell of chemotherapy again and again*, I thought. *And yet again.*

Part Three

LOST

᧖

Chapter 17

TAKING IT ALL OFF

$\wp$

The experts were right: I began losing my hair on day seventeen. I'm not sure when precisely it began. It might have started coming out in my brush that morning or sometime during the day, but by evening, when I took a shower, all of a sudden a pool of water was swirling around my feet. I looked down and saw a massive amount of hair clogging the drain. My hair was so short that I was shocked at how much there was. I couldn't believe what was happening. But I was losing my hair—all of it. Tears began to run down my cheeks, joining the water from the shower.

The next day, more fell out. "It's becoming thinner and thinner," I said to Melanie during a phone call. Each day I gathered clumps of hair from the shower drain and threw them into the garbage. I picked bunches of hair out of my hairbrush. I found tufts all around the house.

"What is that, Alana?" my mother asked one afternoon. She saw me heading to the kitchen garbage.

"I keep wishing this wasn't happening, but it is," I said, showing her the fistful of hair poking out of my hand.

It was tougher and tougher to look in the mirror. The whole thing sucked. I wrote e-mails to close friends describing how I felt, using precisely that word. I would have used much more vulgar ones, but I didn't want to worry anyone and was also worried that the e-mails wouldn't get through.

I often wore a toque for comfort.

"Mommy, take your hat off. We're inside now," Charley said. Rudy tried to pull it off. But I forgot to take it off sometimes, except when I went to bed. One night I even considered leaving it on.

"Greg, can you turn off the ceiling fan?"

"Why?" He turned it on in the winter, too, to keep the air circulating.

"My head gets cold."

One morning while I was standing in the bathroom avoiding my reflection in the mirror, Charley said to me, "You still look beautiful."

I forced myself to look. I ran my hand over my head. *My little Charley.* How could she be so young and so perceptive?

Greg was passing by and heard what she'd said. "You look cool, and you're lucky you have a nice-shaped head."

I stared at myself, harder this time. My scalp was becoming more and more prominent. I don't know if Greg and Charley were trying to make me feel better or if they meant what they said, but I didn't feel beautiful. I wanted to be super strong, to say I didn't care about my looks, but that wasn't true. I did care. Who didn't? I could handle surgery, I could handle vomiting, I could handle not sleeping, but what it turned out I couldn't handle was having my hair fall out.

ℒ

That night I received an e-mail from Monica in response to the update about losing my hair.

Alana,

I am crying for you, your children, your husband and your hair. It truly does suck.

I am crying because you feel sick to your core, because it isn't fair that you have cancer and not only have to feel awful, but now you think you look awful.

I will stop crying, though. I will think of your beautiful children and husband and how lucky they are to be with you. I will smile at the fact that you have courage and enough energy to be mad at losing your hair.

Buy a wig. Feeling good about the way you look is important—it's making the best of the situation.

I am learning that every day I need to thank the earth for being here. I will hug and kiss my family today because of you. You're shedding light on the darkness called cancer, and will make us feel less afraid if we too are forced onto this path.

Thank you.
Monica

Monica's e-mail made me cry. It also made me feel stronger. I called Melanie once I'd wiped away my tears. Greg was out, I had just put the kids to bed, and I couldn't stand it any longer. "I've had enough," I said. "I can't do this anymore. I'm sobbing every time I take a shower, every time I see hair go floating down the drain. Will you buzz the rest of it off?"

She came over right away. "Ready?" she asked, clippers in hand.

"So ready," I said. When I felt the cold metal brushing against my skin,

I felt both depressed and glad. After she was finished, I faced the mirror again. I couldn't help but smile—I looked tough, and I felt tough as well.

"What do you think?" Melanie asked.

"It looks way better buzzed than it did with those stupid uneven clumps. I wish I'd buzzed it after the first strand fell out." I ran my fingers over my scalp. "It feels good. I'm relieved. Although it'll take some time to get used to being bald. But I will."

"Can I?"

"Sure." I bent my head towards her.

Her hands felt warm on my skin, and when I lifted my head up again, I saw she was smiling. "You are going to rock this, Alana."

"I look cool now, don't I?"

"Not just this," she said firmly as she touched my head again.

I thought for a minute. I was going to rock it—the haircut and the struggle. I was feeling more hopeful about that with each passing day.

❧

How would people react to my bald head, especially my immediate family? Greg had always said he thought I was good-looking. What would he think of me with my hair entirely gone? What would my daughter think, especially since she was such a girlie girl? And Rudy—at nine months old, how would he react to the change in my appearance? I put on one of my new *Believe* hats.

"You look good," my mother said.

"Thanks." She never failed to try to make me feel good.

"I can't believe how much colder my head is with no hair at all." I hesitated, and then went on. "Luckily, my eyebrows and eyelashes are intact—small miracles!" I grinned when I felt like doing anything but. I felt like a badly plucked chicken.

"You're lucky I used to lay you on your tummy when you were a baby. That's why your head is so perfectly round. You should thank me!" We both laughed out loud, but she was right. My head was round. Round and almost bald.

Although my head had been shaved, wisps of hair where it hadn't fallen out at the roots were popping up in patches on my head here and there. But by day twenty-one they too fell out.

"It's only hair," people told me. "You look great." Others said, "It'll grow back before you know it." I knew they meant well, were trying to make me feel better, but it didn't help. As a woman, I felt that I was defined by my hair to a great extent—making sure it looked good, brushing it, playing with it, putting it up, curling or straightening it, cutting it, coloring it. I often laughed about the bottles of hair spray I went through as a teenager trying to get my hair "just right." It was so hard first to imagine life without hair, then to have to live that reality.

I began to wear that *Believe* hat constantly during the day. The only time I took it off was to shower. I even began sleeping with it all the time. I didn't expose my head to anyone, even the people I was closest to—my mother, my husband, my children! I just couldn't.

The only person who asked to see my head without a hat was Charley—Greg didn't, neither did my mother. Greg acted as though my having no hair didn't bother him in the least. He didn't treat me any differently because of it, which I was grateful for. But the fact that they didn't want to see it—to see me as I was—tormented me. I knew they were doing it out of love, but I wanted to feel safe revealing myself at my weakest. It would mean I could at last let go, let them take care of me in all my vulnerability.

Only Charley asked. "Okay," I said. "It's your special treat—yours and Rudy's—to see my head, okay?" She looked so surprised. I took my hat off. I felt exposed.

She felt my head. "I love the way it feels."

"I'm so happy you do." I expected her to be scared, and she reacted better than I could have imagined. To her, I was still Mommy. Nothing had changed.

"Thanks, Mommy," she said, pulling her hand away and smiling her beautiful smile.

"I hope my hair will start to grow back by your birthday in March."

"Really?" She reached up and unclipped a flower barrette from her hair. "Here, Mommy, you can wear this next summer."

I almost started crying. "Charley! How lucky am I? That's just what I'll do!"

As for Rudy, I swear he did a double take when he saw me the first time with no hair. Then he wriggled off to wreak havoc as usual, unfazed by my appearance. I don't know why I'd been so worried he'd get upset, too.

"He has so much energy!" I said to Erin one night. "He's so quick, if there were an Olympics for crawling, he'd win gold."

"They never stop, do they?"

"He's getting into everything. He chases me around all the time. When I open the fridge, he tries to crawl into it—one day he got right into it and grabbed a beer. When I open the dishwasher, he goes for it, and when I open the door to go out, there he is."

"Are you getting enough rest?"

"I'm okay." I actually was so tired, but I was trying to keep everything as "normal" as possible for everyone, especially the kids. I was starting to sleep better using Ativan, but it wasn't helping as much as I'd hoped. I'd had that prescription of Ativan since my first night of chemo when I'd started throwing up and had to go to the hospital. "I try to tire Charley and Rudy out during the day so that early in the afternoon we can all get a nap, but usually they end up sleeping while I lie there trying to fall asleep. And just as I start dropping off, they invariably wake up."

"That always happens! You can't sleep when they do."

"If I weren't so busy with them, though, I don't know what I'd do." But I did. I'd end up wallowing in self-pity, because always in the back of my mind was the thought that just as I started to feel better, there would be another treatment and I'd feel like crap again.

<p>

The wig shop called: My wig was ready. I should have been excited, but I wasn't. I was depressed and I felt crappy because of the chemo. Carlo had done an amazing job styling it, though. He helped me to get it in the right spot. Then he placed it on a frame so it would keep its shape and put it in a box. When I got home, I put the box straight in my closet.

I splurged and bought myself a gorgeous soft toque. I'd been wearing the *Believe* hat around the house, but it wasn't as soft on my head as I'd hoped. I figured I could wear this new one for months, but I shouldn't have bothered because the next day, I received a package in the mail. It was a gift from my aunt Audrey, who lived a couple of hours away in Toronto. I called her right away.

"You made all of these?" I asked. She'd sent almost fifteen hats in a rainbow of colors.

"Every one. There are ten for you and extras for Greg and the kids, too."

Then more hats came flooding in from family and friends: handmade toques, thicker ready-made ones—even one that looked like the original sock monkey. I'd be set for the worst of winter, and the timing of my chemo treatments couldn't have been more perfect—it would be easy getting away with wearing a hat all the time, even indoors.

As I stroked one of Aunt Audrey's cozy toques and admired how incredibly soft it was, though, I couldn't help but wonder how long I'd have to go through the hell of living without my hair.

Chapter 18

A NUMBERS GAME

I never realized it until this all happened, but it turns out I am a numbers girl. "Right now I'm 25 percent of the way through chemo, and tomorrow I'll be 37.5 percent through, or 38 percent if you like to round up."

Nina laughed. She was driving me to chemotherapy, and all I could talk about were the percentages I had accomplished.

"I do like to round up—it sounds better," I added. "Thanks again for the *Boobie Brigade* T-shirt." We were both wearing them and planned on rocking the chemo suite.

"They're fun, aren't they?"

"I love them! And I appreciate you coming with me," I said. "When I put all the treatment dates in my calendar, I knew I'd have to get help. Greg wouldn't be able to take all that time off work, and someone had to take care of the kids, too. And when I sent out an e-mail asking for people to drive me to chemotherapy treatments, I didn't know I'd get the kind of response I did."

"What do you mean?"

"I'm a hot ticket! Within an hour, all of the spots were filled. I even had to turn people down—I wanted to make sure Erin and other family members would have the chance to come. I think it will make a difference having people experience it firsthand. But you know that already."

Nina nodded. She'd taken her uncle to JCC for cancer treatment, but sadly he'd passed away. I hoped going back wouldn't be too difficult for her.

"I am glad I can do this for you, Alana," she said.

Nina was such a good friend. Reactions to my diagnosis varied. Some of my friends were scared and backed away, while others—like Nina—dove right in to support me any way they could. I was initially offended that some people couldn't handle it. I couldn't help but think, *If they can't handle it, how on earth will I?* But then I realized that everyone was sensitive to different things, and that they all handled their fear—which is essentially what it was—in different ways, and that I had to be accepting of that. I admired Nina's determination despite the circumstances.

I pushed my seat back, trying to relax. Heading to chemo always made me feel antsy. "It's hard to believe that by the New Year, I'll be 50 percent done. And hopefully onto the less nauseating medicine."

"The next one won't be as bad?"

"Not that way, apparently, but it does come with a whole other whack of side effects."

"Of course," Nina said wryly.

"Wouldn't be chemotherapy without side effects! I'd totally understand why someone would want to play hooky on chemo. I feel great right

Then I realized that everyone was sensitive to different things, and that they all handled their fear—which is essentially what it was—in different ways, and that I had to be accepting of that.

now—like I could run a marathon—but I know that soon I'll feel like an absolute bag of garbage for more than a week. It's hard to go for that reason. You might have to drag me into JCC kicking and screaming," I joked.

"It's terrible that you have to do something so awful, but knowing it's helping makes a difference, doesn't it?"

"Yeah. It's like childbirth that way. It hurts so badly, but you know something good is coming of it."

$\wp$

In the blood lab, I was thrilled to find out that my numbers had improved since the last time, except for my white blood counts. They were a little low but within what was considered a normal range.

"That's great news," I said to Nina as we headed to the chemo suite. I took a number once we got there, and showed it to her, explaining the system. "I think my great blood work is mostly due to Dr. Julia."

"Who's that?" she asked, just as my number was called.

"A chiropractor in Niagara Falls." We walked over to my assigned lounge chair, and I got comfortable. "A friend of mine told me Dr. Julia knows a lot about nutrition, and I wanted to talk to someone about what I was putting in my body, what chemotherapy was doing to me, and how I could improve how I was feeling."

"Makes sense."

"You know me, Nina, if you'd asked me before my diagnosis, I would have said I was fairly healthy. We've always eaten lots of fruits and vegetables, skim milk, fish and lean meat, and we drink plenty of water."

"People even laughed about you making your own laundry soap."

"True! That takes a bit of effort, but honestly, it works well!" It occurred to me how ironic it was that Nina and I were talking about why I made my own soap to avoid toxic chemicals as a nurse inserted an IV needle into me so I could be injected full of toxic chemicals.

"So what did this Dr. Julia have to say?" Nina asked.

"A lot." I'd left her office with a truckload of information. "Her main recommendation was that I eat a plant-based diet and stay away from coffee and alcohol. But I get to drink fruit smoothies every day, too!"

"So that's why you've gone vegan? I knew you had, I just didn't know all the details."

"I'm doing everything I can to beat this." The nurse finished checking my vitals and left, and I shifted in the lounge chair so I could look at Nina more easily. "But it's a big change," I said. "The Dinner Club is in full swing, and I'm finding it incredibly difficult. All that delicious and rich comfort food shows up, and everybody sits there eating it like royalty, while I chomp away on unprocessed greens."

Nina couldn't help but laugh.

"But you won't believe what's happening. Some people have started bringing two dishes on their nights: a regular meal for the family and a vegan meal for me. Everyone has been more amazing than I ever could have imagined." Gabby was stuffing me with food, and so was Adriana. I honestly don't know how she did it. She worked until three P.M. as an educational assistant at the school where I taught, yet came over to our house once a week to bring us food. Then on top of all that, she went to work at a group home where she took care of disabled adults.

I swallowed and couldn't talk for a minute. "I have such incredible friends," I said to Nina.

She touched my hand with the IV, then pulled back all of a sudden.

"Don't worry, they tape it up pretty good," I said. "See?" I waved my hand around and showed her the IV site. "Still intact! I can't help but feel there's a real connection between what I'm eating and how I feel. I went to a bridal shower last weekend and gorged on cheese, meat, sweets—everything. The rest of the evening I felt so uncomfortable. My body seems to be talking to me, even yelling at me sometimes, to give it *good* food. And now that I am, my blood work is reflecting that!"

We high-fived each other.

"I've even decided to try to convert Greg, but he's going to be a hard sell," I said. He was a true carnivore. I wasn't sure he would ever go for it.

The nurse came and checked my vitals again. Everything was great—no nausea, no reactions. Nina was doing okay, too. After the nurse left, she said, "I have a treat for you." She reached down into her bag, pulled out her camera, flicked it on and handed it to me.

I glanced at the screen. "This is amazing, Nina!" She had videotaped the entire hair-shaving party.

"There's more: I got everyone at the school together and recorded messages well before the party."

I couldn't believe it. It was now the middle of December. Among the messages were ones from Melanie, Brody, and other staff and students. I laughed at some; at others my eyes started to well up.

I replayed a message from our librarian, Lorraine. She may have been the kindest woman I'd ever worked with. The kids loved her and so did the staff.

I looked at Nina. She seemed distressed. "What's the matter?"

"About a month after Lorraine taped that message, she was diagnosed with a brain tumor. It's cancer, and they aren't giving her much time."

I closed my eyes. All the feelings I'd had when I was diagnosed resurfaced. "I can't believe it." I didn't know what else to say. Lorraine had been at my party and didn't know at that moment she, too, had cancer. How many other people were walking around with cancer growing inside of them? What was happening when so many people were being diagnosed with this horrible disease? Was it something we were being exposed to? Something we had done? Was I crazy for changing my diet? For making my own laundry soap? Was getting cancer something that was bound to happen from early on because of our genetic makeup?

I was about to find out.

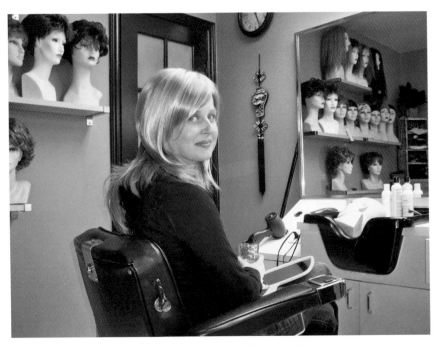

Here I am at the hair studio. I'm not sure I liked the look of this wig—it just wasn't me.

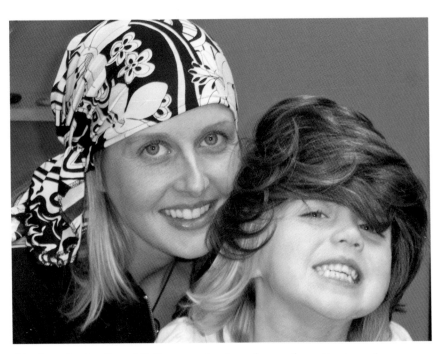

Charley is having fun while I try on a head scarf as an alternative to a wig.

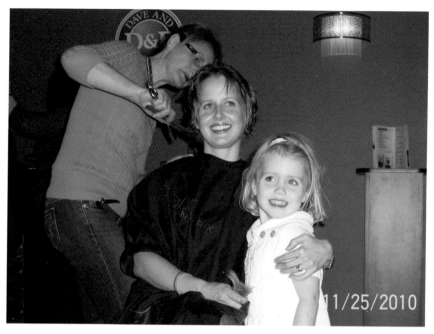

Charley decided to join me while I was getting my hair cut.

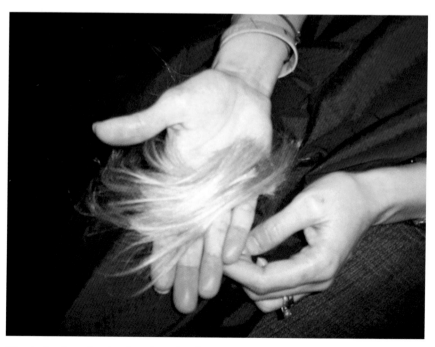

Here's the first chunk of my hair that Lepa cut off.

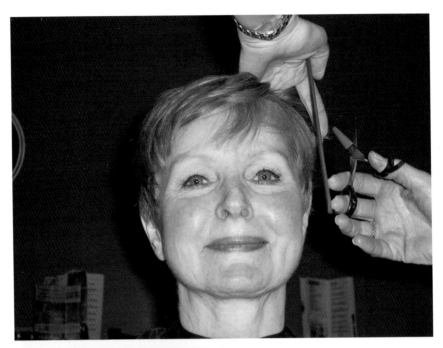

My mother got her hair cut as short as mine. She looks great!

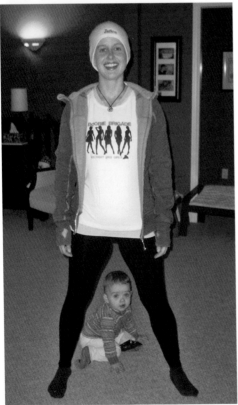

This photo was taken before my third chemo treatment. My hair had completely fallen out by this point, but I was still feeling decent.

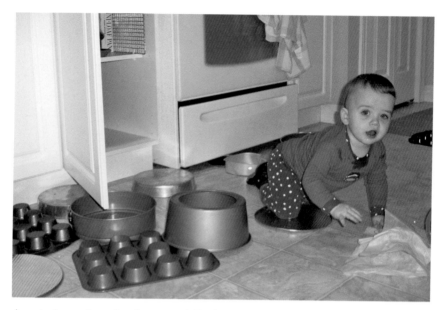

A typical morning often began with Rudy on the rampage in the kitchen, emptying out the cupboards, happy as can be.

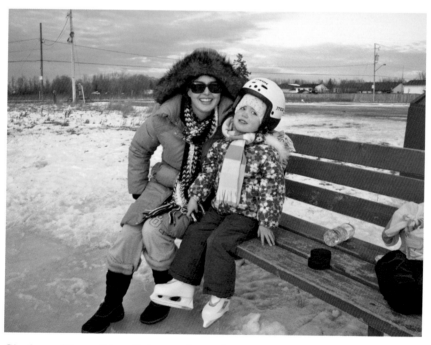

Charley and I are all bundled up at the outdoor ice rink down the road from where we lived.

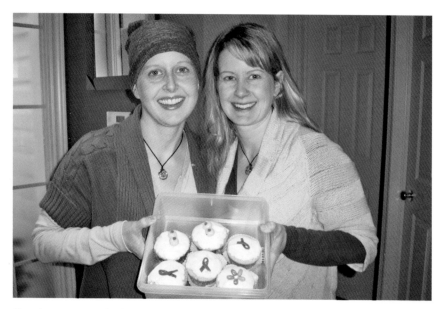

On the morning before I left for my last chemo appointment, my sister, Erin, brought me boobie cupcakes to share with the nurses. Chemo had definitely taken its toll on me—I look more sickly in this photo than I did at any other time.

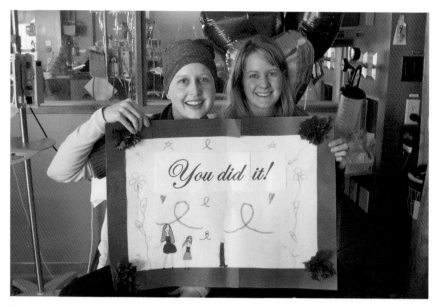

This is a sign my niece and nephew, Erin's kids, made for me to celebrate my last chemo session. I cried. I was happy to be finished but sad there were so many people who weren't close to being done. A small part of me felt ashamed to be celebrating in front of them.

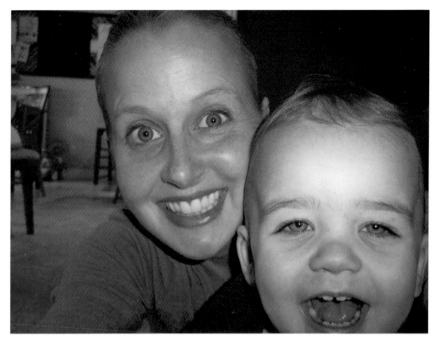

Here's a selfie of Rudy and me at home. My hair was starting to come back, and I was slowly starting to feel better.

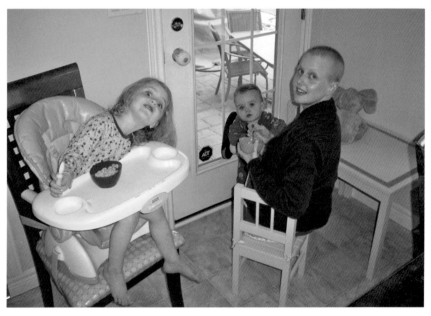

At home with the kids. My hair was getting long enough that I didn't feel the need to wear a toque anymore.

This X-ray of my chest reveals my expanders, metal valves through which saline could be injected into my implants. The expanders gave the X-ray technician a bit of a shock.

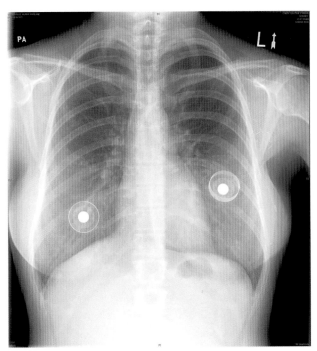

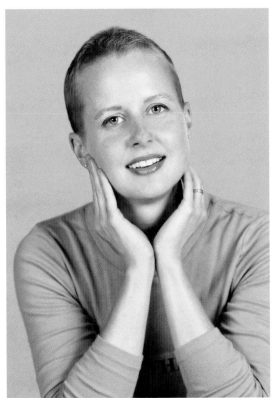

My friend Kim, who was my wedding photographer, felt it was important to document the changes in my appearance. At times the last thing I wanted was to be photographed, but I'm grateful to have these pictures to remind me of the battle I endured and how much stronger I am because of it.

KIM CARTMELL, FOCUS ON YOU PHOTOGRAPHY

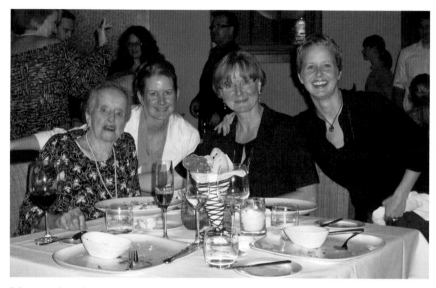

My grandmother, sister, mother and I celebrating my grandmother's ninety-first birthday. This photo is in my living room in a frame with the words "Home is where your story begins." I am proud of being the woman my grandmother and my mother helped me become.

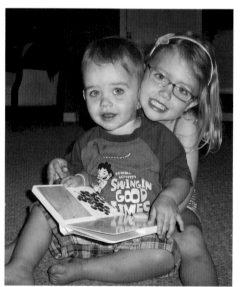

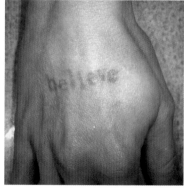

LEFT: My two loves, Charley and Rudy: they are the two reasons I never gave up.
RIGHT: *Believe*—my motto throughout my entire illness. This was stamped on my hand after I dropped the puck at a hockey game to support breast cancer research.

Chapter 19

THE GREAT UNKNOWN

*W*e were all anxious about the results of the genetic testing. But it was Charley I was most concerned for. I couldn't have cared less what the results were for myself—I already had cancer, so testing positive wouldn't change that. But for Charley, the results were crucial.

"What's bugging you?" Nina asked as we waited in the genetic counselor's office. I was anxiously tapping my fingers on the arm of the chair.

"There's so much at stake. This could change things a lot for my kids and my family." I wasn't sure what else to say to help her understand.

"Try not to worry about it until you hear what the counselor has to say."

That was the same kind of thing my mother would say. She and Nina were both right and were both trying to be kind, but it was easier said than done. While I was glad Nina was with me, I wished I'd changed my plans and brought my mother or Erin instead. It's not that I didn't want Nina there, but this was such an important appointment. I shook off any misapprehensions. It was Nina's turn to come with me, and she was the one who'd support me whatever happened. And I was okay sharing everything I found out at any of my appointments with anyone and everyone. I told myself that this would be no different. But we waited for almost ten minutes, and that whole time I couldn't stop shifting in my seat. What would the results be? The door opened and the counselor came in. She was the same one I'd seen the last time.

"Hi, ladies."

"Hi," I said, twisting my fingers together in an attempt to keep still.

She sat down at the desk, glanced at the papers she had in her hand, and then looked at me. "I'm not surprised by the results based on your family history. Although there was some sort of background with your grandmother's sister, in cases where someone is BRCA1 or BRCA2 positive, there's usually a more significant family history of breast cancer—at least three or four people on at least one side of the family tree. For you, the lack of family history was on your side. The test was negative."

Big sigh. Deep breath. Enormous smile.

"Again, based on your lack of family history, I believed it wouldn't be positive, but I'm glad to confirm it. Since you don't have the gene, the risk of developing a new primary breast cancer in the other breast is lowered," she said, pausing and looking at me to make certain I was paying attention. "But it isn't zero. As of right now, the chance is 0.5 to 1 percent per year."

She wasn't telling me anything I didn't already know. When sitting around waiting for results and surgeries, I did a lot of research.

"There are a couple of stipulations," the counselor continued. "First of all, the test results are only 95 percent accurate. The other issue is that although you tested negative for the BRCA1 and BRCA2 mutations, it's possible there may be other mutations you could have, ones that scientists simply haven't put a name to yet."

I didn't want to think about even more risks, but it seemed I had to.

"In other words, you could be a carrier for BRCA3 or BRCA4 or some further mutation that hasn't yet been identified."

"But as far as you can say right now, my situation is just attributable to bad luck?"

The counselor nodded. That was as far as she would go.

I had no definitive answer as to how I'd ended up with cancer. No way of knowing if I could have done something to prevent it. I would always have questions. I knew my frustration was obvious from the counselor's reaction.

"You do have the option of revisiting the results every couple of years. There is a chance that someone could discover a new genetic mutation. It's not to say that you don't have one, it just might not be discovered yet. We could retest your blood to see if there have been any new breakthroughs," she said patiently. "But it's up to you."

I thanked her, and we left. "The numbers are a lot lower, but not low enough for me," I said to Nina as we made our way to the parking lot. "After twenty years, my risk of recurrence would still be about 20 percent. That's too high. I don't ever want to go through this again."

"What will you do?"

"The doctors have decided I need chemo and one breast removed. I've decided that to totally remove the risk, I'm going to have both breasts removed." I wasn't sure if Nina was shocked or not, but in the same way that I felt empowered after shaving my head, I felt empowered by my decision. It was a no-brainer. I felt almost happy. But in terms of the genetic results, I was most happy for everyone else. My being negative meant my daughter, mother and sister—basically every female relative of mine—could breathe a sigh of relief. It didn't mean that they would never get breast cancer, but it did mean that their risk of getting it was significantly lower.

There were concerns, though, raised by the possibility of future tests for unknown mutations. Charley wouldn't be able to have genetic screening done until she was eighteen, and even if I did test positive for something, that didn't necessarily mean she would. Would I cause myself years of unnecessary worry if I had further tests? Would a positive test make me feel that I'd found the answer to my particular cancer? I couldn't stop thinking. My negative result only led to more and more unknowns.

Chapter 20

NESTING

$\mathcal{P}$

N *esting is something* women apparently do before they have a baby. Their subconscious triggers it, telling them to get ready, so a woman who's nesting will typically do an incredible amount of housework, and that's a sign labor is imminent. What probably happens is that the sheer intensity of all that housework precipitates labor. It's a classic example of which comes first: the chicken or the egg?

I had never experienced nesting with Charley—she surprised us by arriving four weeks early—or with Rudy, because even though he came eleven days late, I felt so much like a beached whale that I wasn't able to do much of anything. After the hell I went through after my first infusion of chemotherapy, things improved somewhat, and I usually started feeling better after about a week following each treatment. It occurred to me that I was slowly beginning a pattern of nesting behavior, although I didn't realize it right away. I simply wanted to get as many of the normal day-to-day tasks done while I could.

The "nesting" would begin on day 10 or 11 after each chemo session. I'd start frantically catching up on everything—doing multiple loads of laundry, grocery shopping, clearing up the toy "maze" the kids had invariably built, vacuuming, organizing the massive number of books in Charley's room, changing bedsheets, paying bills, and responding to e-mails I'd neglected. My mother was an immense help, but she couldn't do everything—she had her own household to look after—and I was anxious to finish whatever I could while I'd have those few good days before the next infusion and round of nausea and vomiting, and I was out of commission.

"Are you sure I can't go get the groceries?" Mom asked one day.

"If you don't mind staying here to watch the kids, I'll go. I'm starting to get a little stir-crazy." I always went outdoors with the kids no matter how I was feeling, so they'd burn off some energy, but running errands would be different. I needed a break from the kids and some me time.

"No, you go!" she said, practically pushing me out the door once she heard that.

I knew she'd understand. My outing didn't last long—I got tired of the awkwardness of being around people who stared at me. Regardless of where I went, I felt as though they looked at me with pity. That may all have been in my head. I wore a toque so no one would know I was bald, but I felt as though they could tell. The staring made me angry, but I kept it to myself. *It's just how people are*, I thought. It did feel good to get out, though. I was determined that I would do it again.

I also got back into my evening routine of going for walks around the block as a de-stressor—something I'd started before I had cancer, once the kids were in bed, since I wasn't much of a "sit on the couch and watch TV" person. It was the dead of winter, but I'd bundle up, crank up the volume on my iPod, and go around the block to get fresh air and clear my mind. I'd keep going until I was fatigued, sometimes for two hours if I was up to it. A few nights after I started this routine again, I got home and Greg was lying on the couch watching TV. "The exercise is so fantastic for my sleep," I said, pulling off my scarf and shaking the snow from it.

"You look good."

I glanced in the mirror. I did look good—my eyes were bright and my cheeks were all pink. Looking at me at that moment, nobody would have guessed I was ill, except for the lack of hair. "It's great when I can get in a walk like this. Some nights, especially now that I'm getting closer to the next treatment, I don't even need to take an Ativan or Zopiclone to have a good sleep." It was a vast improvement. I often didn't sleep well, particularly during the first part of the chemotherapy cycle.

"I know," Greg joked.

I was sure my tossing and turning were keeping him up at night, but he didn't say anything more. "I can't help but think more and more about percentages," I said, collapsing onto the couch beside him and recalling the conversation I'd had with Nina.

"What do you mean?"

"I'll be 50 percent done with chemo. As long as I know that with each treatment I'm getting closer and closer to the end, everything seems bearable. Even the nausea."

"Really?" I could hear the skepticism in his voice. He'd been there for everything and knew what I'd gone through.

"Really. I can't believe I'm almost halfway through. I feel like I can make it now." With that, lying safe beside him, I promptly fell asleep.

$\mathcal{P}$

Melanie took me to my next round of chemo. Since it was my fourth and last AC treatment, to celebrate she brought a picnic basket packed with gourmet goodies: smoked salmon, gourmet crackers, Ezekiel Bread, and homemade hummus, spinach and roasted eggplant dips, and salsa, as well as figs and sweets. In addition to being handy with hair clippers, she was also an amazing cook.

"Everyone's looking at us," she whispered to me in the waiting room.

"It's your basket," I said. "They're envious." We offered everyone some but didn't get any takers—people were too kind to dig into our bounty.

"They must be trying to cram more patients into the suite than usual," I said as our wait dragged out. "The chemo suite is closed part of the week for the Christmas holidays." But the time provided us with the perfect opportunity to enjoy Melanie's feast. I looked around the waiting room as we ate. There were a couple of new patients. I knew they were rookies—I recognized them by their quilts. I remembered how I'd felt when I'd first begun this journey and felt terrible knowing what they were heading into. It was hard to believe I wasn't a newbie anymore, but I was glad I'd come this far.

"Good riddance to AC," I said, and Melanie and I toasted each other with our bottles of water.

The holidays were usually crazy, spent running around town from house to house, visiting relatives, and eating turkey dinner after turkey dinner. I loved that, but this year, Christmas was different from every other.

"I don't want to miss any chemo treatments," I said to Greg. "And you know what it's like during the holidays—the first thing everyone wants to do is hug and kiss everyone else, and people always seem to get sick. I don't want to get sick and I don't want the kids to, either." I had visions of one of us ending up with a fever and having to run to the emergency department. Not my idea of fun over Christmas.

We decided the best way to stay healthy was to avoid as many people as we could, so we stayed home as much as possible. Charley didn't realize anything had changed—she was too young, and so was Rudy. Christmas Eve, I made dinner, and after that, we took the kids for a ride to see the light show at Niagara Falls. It was always such a spectacular event, and with all that had been going on, none of us had had a chance to go. The kids both fell asleep in the car on the way back. "The excitement was a little too much," I said to Greg with a grin. When we got home, we woke Charley up so she could leave out cookies for Santa, then tucked her and Rudy into bed.

Christmas morning, Charley woke us up. "I want to see if Santa ate the cookies, Mommy," was the first thing she said before running out. We got up and followed, after getting Rudy from his room.

"Mommy, he left half a cookie for me," Charley shouted.

I had to smile at Greg. "She hasn't even noticed the presents under the tree, she's so excited about Santa!" There was a knock at the door.

"Mom, Dad!" Their arms were full of presents. Her mouth covered with crumbs, Charley ran over to hug them while they were standing in the doorway. "Charley, let them in."

"Presents!"

"You'll have to wait to open those. Breakfast first."

I steered everyone to the dining room, and Mom helped me in the kitchen while Greg and Dad kept the kids busy.

"You okay with all this, Alana?"

"I'm fine, Mom." And I was. After that first disastrous visit and a little coaching, my dad had become more upbeat, at least in front of me. I was happy to have him and my mother over for a small celebration. "Mom, can you take these out?" I handed her the Baileys coffees I'd made, then followed with a fruit tray and croissants. Charley started squirming before we'd even begun eating, and I gave in.

"Go downstairs and wait by the tree, Charley, we'll be there in a minute. But don't open anything yet!"

She pushed back her chair and ran out, and Rudy tried toddling after her.

"I may have spoiled the kids a little more with presents this year," I said to my mother. "Probably because I wanted to make up for some of the chaos they've had to go through." I couldn't help but think after I'd said that, *I wonder how many more Christmases I have left?*

"You have every right to do that. I spoiled them a bit more this year, too."

"I don't want them to feel different, Mom. I just don't want them to be affected by this."

"Alana, you and the kids are all going to be stronger because of this. I know it," she said as she picked up the fruit tray and carried it down. The rest of us followed with our unfinished coffees, and the kids began tearing into the presents.

"Charley's getting to the age where she is starting to get it, isn't she?" I said to Greg. "It's exciting to see."

"Rudy's still happy playing with wrapping paper and empty boxes."

"It's true!" They had a blast and so did we. After all the presents had been opened and my mother had helped me clean up the kitchen and some of the wrapping paper—"Let's leave some out for Rudy," I said—my parents were off.

"We don't want to miss the Christmas morning fun at Erin's," Mom said.

I knew the subtext was that they didn't want to tire me out.

After lunch and a nap for the kids, Greg's mother came over to spend the rest of the day with us. His father had passed away a couple of years earlier in an accident, and I missed him. He'd been the best father-in-law anyone could ask for, and I wished he could have been around. Christmas was a tough time for all of us without him, but especially for Greg's mother, and we were happy to have her over. But she'd changed after Greg's father passed away, becoming more distant, especially since I'd been diagnosed. She didn't want to talk about my cancer or treatments, and whenever she was around, it was as if there were a big elephant in the room. I imagined that if Greg's father had been there, everything would have been much more open. He would even have joked around with me. That was his way—relaxed and funny. Greg and I didn't talk about that, though. He'd been so affected by his father's death—probably more than even I knew—and I wasn't sure I wanted to go there.

On Boxing Day we ventured out to my parents'. Normally they'd have a houseful of people, but my mother had promised, "It will only be a small gathering," and it was. We had an intimate dinner for six.

"This is so relaxing, Mom. I hope you don't mind that it's smaller," I said.

"Not at all. This is actually quite nice!"

I looked around the table. Charley was happily stuffing her face with turkey, and Greg was heaping his plate with a second helping of stuffing. Rudy's face was covered with bits of mashed potato. It was perfect. Despite our sticking close to home, Christmas had proven to have been fantastic—different, for sure, but wonderful. In fact, probably the best Christmas ever, and Greg was happy with how low-key it was as well.

I finished off another spoonful of potatoes. "I think I'm starting to know how you feel on a daily basis," I said to Greg.

"What do you mean?"

"I feel queasy, but as long as I have food in my stomach that seems to help, so I'm trying to keep eating all the time."

He laughed.

"It's true! I'm positive I've never eaten so much in my life!" I couldn't possibly eat more, nor could anyone else—even Greg. Mom and I started to clear the table, and I said, "I feel great. I even managed to stick to my diet by eating all the vegetables."

She smiled, but waited for me to continue as we went into the kitchen—I think she knew I had something on my mind. "The Taxol part of chemo starts soon, and I don't know if the diet will work as well with it."

"But the nausea will be gone, right?" she asked.

"Right," I said, knowing I didn't sound very confident. I'd talked to women at JCC and discovered that while some found Taxol more bearable than AC, others found it less.

"Don't worry about something you don't know about yet," Mom said.

It was a refrain I would have to learn to live by, I told myself. I had no idea how I would be affected. Nobody did.

Chapter 21

MOVING, MOVING, MOVING . . . ON

I was anxious and leery about the amount of drugs I needed to take before my first Taxol session. I'd already been taking two dexamethasones per day for the first three days after each of my earlier chemo sessions to help with nausea, but for this second half of chemotherapy, I had to take ten (ten!) before each appointment—five pills twelve hours before and another five pills six hours before, even if that meant waking up in the middle of the night—since the drug was a steroid and would help minimize the high risk of reactions.

"They make me edgy, and I can't help but feel I'm going to be outside running laps around the block in the middle of the night instead of sleeping," I said to Erin when she called one afternoon. "Even days after I took that cycle of two pills, I had a hard time getting a good night's sleep because of the lingering effects."

"Is there nothing you can do?"

"The only thing that works is my nightly walks. And I've cracked out a few old yoga videos I found in the basement." During pregnancy and when the kids were infants, I'd found it hard to stay as active as I wanted, so I'd gotten exercise videos I could work out to without leaving the house. "I've been trying to do those close to bedtime, but I sometimes need to take an Ativan before bed to get to sleep, although I try not to rely on it that much."

The first night I had to take the increased dose of dexamethasone, I ate a bowl of cereal at ten P.M.—I had to take the pills with juice or food—even though we'd had some of Adriana's delicious food for dinner and I wasn't hungry. Then I took the required five pills and got ready for bed. "I cannot wait to have all these drugs out of my system," I said to Greg irritably and crawled in beside him. I wanted to try to get any sleep I could before the pills took effect and left me lying wide awake, staring at the ceiling. The next thing I knew, I heard a buzzing noise.

"You slept!"

I turned over. "I know!" I was as surprised as Greg. It was already four A.M. I lay back for a moment, relishing the thought that I'd made it right through the night. "I already feel a bit edgy, though." It was an odd sensation. "Not tired, which is great, but different from my usual self." I felt fidgety and impatient. Like I wanted to leap out of bed to get moving—and keep moving. This wasn't normal at all, and I was sure it was the dexamethasone.

"I'm going to get up and go on the computer. Don't worry, I'll try to not wake up the kids!"

"Okay," Greg said. "Do what you need to do." I got dressed and made my way to the kitchen. I swallowed the next five of the dexamethasone pills with some juice. I decided I was going to take advantage of the brief time to myself. I headed to the basement and did some online banking, checked out Facebook posts, then googled breast cancer statistics. I became so immersed in the numbers, I didn't realize it was already six A.M. I quietly ran upstairs to shower. By the time I got out and made my way back out, my mother was up. She'd heard the kids moving about and was keeping them occupied.

"Hey, Mom!"

"Hi, honey."

"I'm so glad you decided to come the night before my appointments." I looked out the window. "You never know what the weather's going to be like." I got the kids settled at the kitchen table, made myself a smoothie, and was just starting to give Mom a rundown on who needed to do what during the day when I heard a knock at the door.

Charley ran and opened it before I could. "Uncle Doug!"

"Hey, your chauffeur for the day is here!" I could hear my brother-in-law call out.

"I'm coming," I said to him. "Just let me get my smoothie." I kissed the kids and my mom, grabbed the smoothie and a lunch I'd packed, and we were off.

"How are you?" Doug asked once we pulled out onto the road.

"Good. Well, better than I have been. I'll have to see how today goes."

"Something different about today?"

"I'm starting another drug."

I wondered if he was worried about my throwing up all over the place.

"You'll tell me how to get to where we are going, right?"

"Of course."

I was happy to be spending the day with Doug, but didn't feel very talkative, so we didn't chat much more. I knew he wouldn't mind. I was most nervous about the possibility of a reaction but didn't want to admit that, and certainly not to my brother-in-law. Sharing what I was experiencing—even with the people closest to me—wasn't getting any easier, and I didn't want anyone to feel bad

Sharing what I was experiencing—even with the people closest to me— wasn't getting any easier, and I didn't want anyone to feel bad for me. I also didn't want them to think that everything was always about me, either.

for me. I also didn't want them to think that everything was always about me, either. More often than not of late my conversations with people *were* all about me, so when I had a chance to talk about something else—or not talk at all—it was a relief.

My blood work was even better this time. I felt great about that, as though it was confirmation that my diet really was working. As I pressed the button in the elevator to head up to the chemo suite, I thought, *If it is, then maybe I do have power over something.*

When my number was called and we entered the suite, I was surprised to be led to a stretcher. "Before, I always got one of those," I said to Doug, pointing at a lounge chair. I'd told everyone about them, how sitting in them was like being in someone's comfy rec room. I could tell Doug was taken aback by the whole situation. Everyone with me reacted the same way—I could see it in their eyes. This wasn't the sort of thing they saw every day. Doug tried to keep me smiling as if it were his job to make me feel comfortable. He didn't realize I was used to it and that I was usually the one who tried to make the people who came with me feel comfortable.

The nurse who was going to be helping me overheard my comment. "You'll be here such a long time, we give you a stretcher so you can fall asleep," she said.

I did know that instead of forty-five minutes for the AC infusion I'd been used to, the Taxol infusion would take three to four hours—they infused the drug slowly because of the increased risk of a reaction—but I hadn't realized that would change things.

The nurse handed me a Benadryl. "That's a precaution against a reaction. And the stretcher's not just for naps. If you do have a reaction, it'll be easier for us to treat you if you're lying down."

I got settled, and the nurse started the IV, then sat beside me to monitor my vital signs. I kept looking at my watch.

"You okay?" Doug asked.

He looked so concerned. "Yeah," I lied. "I'm fine." I knew the first ten minutes were crucial in terms of a reaction. Those ten minutes took forever. I kept expecting something dramatic to happen—hives, chills, fever. I was anticipating it. The nurse watched me intently, waiting for something to happen, which only increased my fears. What worried me most was the knowledge that when there was a reaction, it was fairly severe. Would I have an anaphylactic reaction? I tried calming myself down by breathing deeply. It didn't work.

"Are you having trouble breathing?" the nurse asked.

"No."

"Do you feel flushed at all?"

"No."

"Are you feeling in any way different than you did before the infusion began?"

"No."

The questions continued, each making me more anxious. After several more minutes of interrogation, I was pleased and surprised to have passed the ten-minute mark.

"Great. The chance of having a reaction after ten minutes is unlikely, and the chance of having a reaction at your next appointment is even unlikelier."

When it was clear that I was going to be okay, the nurse left us alone, just Doug, the Taxol and me.

I relaxed. One less thing I needed to worry about. I even started to feel sleepy enough to think about taking a nap. The only thing I was now worried about was if I would drool in front of Doug.

Chapter 22

GRASPING AT STRAWS

ℒ

B*y the Thursday* after my first Taxol treatment, I was still feeling good—much better than I had during the AC treatments. A slight head-ache, but no nausea. And I was energetic. It was a huge relief. I knew some side effects could appear, and apparently one in three women had such achy bones they needed Tylenol 3 or even Percocet, but I was keeping my fingers crossed. I had tried Percocet after my lumpectomy, but it was so strong that I didn't use too much of it. I had also heard it was highly addictive, so that was another reason I wanted to stay away from it. Was it possible after the hell of my first four AC treatments that I would have a better-than-average experience going forward?

Whatever was going on, I was determined to take advantage of feeling good. I pulled my wig out of my closet and tried it on again, but realized right away how itchy and hot it felt—the hot flashes didn't help. I thought the wig looked funny, too, not natural at all. In a weird way, I also think I was getting used to having no hair, and I was already so self-conscious at that point that I didn't want to make things any worse. I packed the wig away and got out the plans for our new house.

A couple of years earlier, Greg and I had started house hunting, or rather property hunting. We'd built the house we were living in, and loved it, but when we put a pool in the backyard, we'd very much limited the space there. We knew we could probably make money selling the house, so we started looking for property to build on. We'd seen a few one-acre lots, but they either weren't in a desirable area, needed a lot of work, or were just too expensive. We were starting to think we weren't going to be able to find exactly what we wanted.

One day I visited Susanne, and told her about our dilemma.

"Have you ever looked at that place?" she asked, pointing out the window to a vacant piece of farmland nearby. She and her husband lived on a giant piece of land not far from us.

"It's not for sale."

"Neither was ours when we bought it. Years ago, a lot of the property in this area was owned by a guy who lived in Germany. He bought hundreds of acres, severed it into smaller portions, then sold them off to other Germans under the premise that the properties were close to Niagara Falls. It might be worth looking into."

"But it's not close to Niagara Falls."

"I know, silly, but when you live in Germany, this *is* really close."

We laughed, but Susanne had piqued my interest. I tracked down the name of the owner through public records, and in the wee hours of the night, to account for the time change, tried calling. After three wrong numbers, I was about to give up, but finally got the son of the owner. He told me someone had offered 40,000 euros for the land. I made a counteroffer for higher. I felt rather giddy about that.

"Let me speak to my father and get back to you."

The next day, I got a phone call. They had accepted my offer. I had just purchased a thirty-five-acre piece of land for under $70,000 Canadian. I was ecstatic.

"They accepted my offer," I told Greg when he got home.

"You're kidding!"

"I've already called the bank and the lawyer and he's working on the paperwork before they can change their minds."

"What a steal!" he said. "Nice work!"

I knew that was only the beginning, though. I looked at the house plans; we were still working on them. As I glanced around our current house, it was hard to believe we'd be leaving it. We'd created so many memories in it. Brought both of our children home from the hospital to it. Spent every birthday and Christmas in it. But I'd also been diagnosed with cancer there. I jotted some notes on the plans. Maybe moving would allow us to make a fresh start, put some things behind us.

It was also time to make decisions about yet another drug, metformin, which was undergoing clinical trials. Margo at CAREpath had called to tell me about the trial. From my very first talk with her, she had suggested asking the team at JCC if there were clinical trials I would qualify for.

"The idea is daunting," I'd told my mother. "I'll be acting as a lab rat, in essence." I had let Margo know I didn't want to participate in chemotherapy trials. "I want to be given drugs that work. I don't want to mess around with my life." But the metformin study sounded promising. Honestly, anything that showed any sign of hope would have sounded promising.

Both my oncologist and surgeon had told me that because of the particular kind of cancer I had—triple negative—if there was going to be a recurrence, it would happen within the first two years. Thus if I made it to three years, it was highly unlikely there would be any recurrence at all. From my research, I knew that many women who, unlike me, had estrogen receptor positive breast cancer could receive drugs called aromatase inhibitors like Herceptin and tamoxifen, which acted as estrogen bodyguards—they prevented estrogen from feeding cancer. Those women were able to take the drugs for only five years following chemotherapy, but that was like a "get out of jail free" card they could use to gain five years without a recurrence. For me and other triple negative patients, there was no such thing. I would just be sent on my merry way.

Margo explained when we talked, though, that doctors had noticed that cancer patients who had Type 2 diabetes and were also on metformin—a drug used to control and keep insulin levels low—had lower recurrence rates. The clinical trial would look at whether metformin could decrease or affect the ability of breast cancer cells to grow and whether metformin would work with other therapies to prevent cancer from recurring. Given that situation, I was keen to find out more, and naturally I met with the clinical trials nurse, a woman named Helen. I had a lot of questions.

"Do the diabetes patients have lower recurrence rates because of the metformin or because their insulin levels are low?"

"Recurrence rates are lower because of low insulin levels," she said, "which are made low because of the drug."

"Can a person achieve low insulin levels with diet and exercise alone?"

"Absolutely."

I stared at her. Essentially I could participate in a clinical trial and take metformin once a day for the first month, and then twice a day for the next five years, or I could eat the right food, exercise, and avoid sugar to keep my insulin levels low without the help of a drug. I was puzzled. I wanted to do everything possible to reduce my chances of a recurrence, but the last thing I wanted was to take even more drugs.

For the next three days, all I could think about was metformin. I asked my mom her opinion, I asked Greg, I researched it on the internet, and I struggled with the decision. Should I take part in the trial? Was it worth it? Soon, however, I would forget all about the trial.

Chapter 23

WHAT A PAIN

P

After three days of feeling glorious, my legs began to ache—a dull, insidious pain that is a nasty side effect of Taxol. I was devastated. I was clearly delusional to think I was out of the woods, that nothing could be worse than the vomiting and nausea associated with the AC part of chemotherapy. I thought I had avoided the side effects altogether. What a cruel trick my brief spell of wellness had been.

> I was devastated. I was clearly delusional to think I was out of the woods.

Later that night, as I lay in bed trying to fall sleep—already difficult due to all the steroids—I began to feel the oddest sensation in my legs in addition to the aching. Like they wanted to go for a walk without me. Although they weren't moving spontaneously, the only thing that made me more comfortable was to move them. I couldn't escape that feeling—it was what I imagined restless legs syndrome must be like. No matter how hard I tried to keep quiet so I could fall asleep—and because I was trying to not wake up poor Greg—I couldn't stop moving my legs. I was near tears I was so exhausted.

By morning I felt like a Raggedy Ann doll that had lost most of its stuffing. The sensations in my entire body seemed heightened, and although the number of bones and muscles in my body obviously hadn't changed, I felt as though I could feel exactly where they all were. Worse, I could swear that my bones were being crushed over and over again. Usually I considered myself able to tolerate pain well. If relief from pain was ever necessary, I popped a Tylenol. When it came to what I was suffering with Taxol, though, Tylenol didn't even touch the pain. Neither did Motrin. I took a Tylenol 3—I knew it had codeine in it—but after waiting anxiously for two hours for the aches to subside even a little, I realized this wasn't doing a thing, either. Could Taxol actually be the more evil chemotherapy drug? I was getting so cranky, I felt sorry for everyone around me. I was sure I was a real treat to live with.

Charley didn't notice. "Mommy, can we go outside and play in the snow?" she asked. The snow had piled up from a snowfall the night before. We all got bundled up, Rudy included, and went out. I grabbed a shovel for myself and a smaller plastic one for Charley and went to work. Within an hour the driveway and sidewalk were shoveled and my body was fatigued. That helped a little with the achiness and the restlessness of my legs, and Charley and Rudy had fun.

I knew I couldn't keep moving all day, though. I needed something to take the pain away and I couldn't get another prescription right away from my doctor; it was a Saturday, so I was out of luck. "Greg, could you please, please go to the drugstore to get me something for the pain? I can't take it anymore."

"Absolutely, but what's going to work if Tylenol 3 doesn't?"

"Aleve. Get Aleve." I didn't have a clue, but I was desperate. I knew it was a nonsteroidal anti-inflammatory drug, and when I'd had menstrual cramps, it was the only thing that took the pain away. When Greg got home, I practically tore the bag out of his hands and gulped down the pill as soon as I could get it out of the bottle. My instincts were right. After about an hour, the pain subsided. Unfortunately, after I took the Aleve, my nose started to bleed. Not drastically, but enough that every time I had to blow my nose I started going into another room so the kids wouldn't see it.

That's what I did: Throughout this whole thing, I never allowed them to see anything that might make them scared or nervous. As exhausted, nauseous, scared or anxious as I might have been, I faked it in front of my family, my friends, everyone. I didn't want anyone to worry about me.

And I had to admit, it was a bonus that Aleve didn't give me the awful constipation Tylenol 3 did. As crazy as it sounds, it would sometimes be three days before I'd be able to go to the bathroom properly if I took it. My digestive system was sensitive as it was—unless I followed a fairly regular diet, things got totally off schedule. None of the other drugs seemed to have the same effect, but I had learned to have a gentle over-the-counter laxative on hand, just in case. And with all of the different drugs being thrown my way, I never knew what to expect.

Once I lay down, the pain became unbearable. So during the day I kept moving as much as possible. With the kids around, I didn't have much of a choice—I wanted to play with them, and they wanted to play with me, so I just sucked it up and got through it, day by day. Plus, to be honest, I was too obsessive about things like toys all over the floor to watch them pile up. I was definitely slower at everything, though.

Only two other things were helping me get through Taxol. The first was exercise. It strengthened and stretched my muscles, which seemed to ease the pain, and it also tired me out so that by bedtime I could fall asleep. When most people cursed a heavy snowfall, I welcomed blizzard-like conditions: powering through the drifts exhausted me even more. Some nights, before bedtime, I'd get out our old wooden sled and take the kids for rides around and around the block. They loved it, invariably screaming, "Again, again!" each time we neared our driveway.

The second thing that helped was yoga, which I had recently

rediscovered in a desperate attempt to help with sleep and found incredibly relaxing. There were times when I didn't feel like exercising—ironically, I felt too tired to work out so I could fall asleep—and I always had a million things on my mind (the dishes in the sink, the laundry in the dryer, the toys on the floor—everything else that I felt "needed" to be done), but the prospect of being able to sleep was great motivation.

All that wasn't enough. Never in my life had I felt that kind of pain, and never in my life had there not been some sort of medication to get rid of it. Desperate, I turned to Dr. Julia once again.

"Take L-glutamine," she said. "It will help prevent neuropathy, which is the tingling and numbness you've been feeling, and will protect your gastrointestinal tract from the effects of the chemotherapy drugs."

I bought some right away. The supplement did seem to take the edge off the achiness, so I decided to keep taking it for the rest of the treatments. I let my oncologist know, and she was okay with it. Frantic at night, though, I sprayed topical muscle relaxant onto my calves and feet, hoping to numb them, but that was pointless. Sleeping pills were useless. There were three more treatments left, and I was resigned to the fact that the first week after each treatment, no matter how much exercise or yoga I did or what drugs or supplements I took, would remain very uncomfortable.

I took a deep breath and shook my shoulders to relax them. *No problem!* I told myself. *I've already come this far. What will three more treatments take? Besides, with the number of appointments filling my calendar, time will fly by. Before I know it, chemotherapy will be over.* But even as I thought that, I could feel myself tensing up again. I knew that the end couldn't come soon enough.

Part Four

WILL I MAKE IT?

Chapter 24

DISTRACTION

*C*harley and Rudy were handling the whole cancer thing beautifully. In fact, they were handling it so well that the fact that I had cancer wasn't stopping them from doing anything. It was nice to have at least two people in my life who didn't look at me with pity. On the other hand, since they had no pity, they didn't treat me with any special consideration at all.

One morning I heard a crash.

"Rudy, what are you doing?" I called out as I ran over to the kitchen doorway. He was playing his usual game—empty a cupboard, move on to the next, and pull everything out of that—and was chucking things on the floor. This time it was baking sheets, but anything was a target—glass lids, bowls, baking pans, even my grandmother's huge cast-iron pan. "Put that back," I said. He was holding a muffin tin and looking at me with a gleeful smile. He was almost a year old and was turning into the "boy" everyone said he would. I definitely wasn't used to that. Charley had been such an easy toddler. If Rudy got the chance, he'd also take things from the kitchen and throw them down the stairs or put them under the couch in the living room, then take books or toys from the living room and put them into the now-empty kitchen cupboards.

I scooped him up. "Stay still," I said as he tried squirming out of my arms while I attempted to shove a pan back into its place. He managed to scramble down just as the phone rang.

"Hey, it's me," Greg said. "I wanted to call to say hi and see how things are going."

"I've already tidied the floor three times," I said, "and I know the rest of my day is going to consist of exactly the same thing over and over again."

"Just leave it. I'll pick things up when I get home."

"I'm losing my mind." I started bawling. Although I knew that Greg's intentions were good, it seemed to me as though he didn't get what I was going through or know how to sympathize with me—I couldn't handle everything and a messy house on top of it all.

That weekend, he helped me install baby locks on all the cupboards. Meanwhile, Charley was starting to say no to me, and she wasn't shy about it. She was almost four years old and thought she knew everything and could do anything. She did make me laugh a lot, though. One day she decided to wear the new knee-high black boots she'd gotten, but no pants, and she danced around the living room with Buster, her stuffed rabbit toy. Another day, Mom and I could hear her talking. We peeked around the corner and she had her toy phone up to her ear.

"She's talking to her imaginary friend," I said.

"What is she saying?" Mom said.

"Shh, I can't hear." We inched closer.

Charley started talking louder. She was having an intense conversation with Dora the Explorer! Mom and I both looked at each other and had to back out of the room before we burst out laughing.

My entire life had become scheduled to the nth degree, and chasing the kids around was the least of my day-to-day worries. My calendar was jam-packed, from taking medications at certain times, to ensuring that the kids made it to the usual playdates, school events and other things, to getting to my own appointments. Anything to do with cancer stood out, though. I drew a rectangle around the dates of any of those appointments, and there were a lot of rectangles on the calendar. The next one was a meeting with a radiation oncologist on January 17 to discuss whether I'd need radiation.

"I'll do it if I have to," I said to Greg. "But I'm hoping he says I don't need it. The less I have to undergo, the better."

"You've been through a lot already."

I knew radiation could burn my skin. That scared the hell out of me. Again, though, I didn't voice my fears. I simply couldn't.

I also had meetings scheduled with two plastic surgeons to discuss options for breast reconstruction. I was having an entire part of my body removed, and I wanted to get more than one opinion. My mother and I both agreed that was important. The more information I had, the easier it would be to make an educated decision about which surgeon to use and what type of breast-reconstruction surgery would be the better option.

"I'm nervous, but also excited," I said to Mom one day when we were playing with the kids. "This will be one step closer to being healed and healthy again. I feel as though I've started looking at women's breasts in a whole new way," I confessed and picked up a ball Rudy had rolled my way. "I mean, what should mine look like? What will they look like after the fact?" I squeezed the ball. Would my new breasts feel like this? Would everyone be able to tell they weren't real?

"You have to make the decision, Alana."

I sighed. "I do know that the typical wait for a consultation with both surgeons is eight

"I feel as though I've started looking at women's breasts in a whole new way," I confessed. . . . "I mean, what should mine look like?"

months and about a year and a half for surgery. But that's for elective surgery."

"That's a long time." Mom sounded so surprised.

"Turns out having cancer does have some perks," I said wryly. "But I
have no idea what to ask either of the surgeons. Should I ask to see their
work? Surely they must have pictures?" Other than that, I was mystified. It
was such a major decision. How would I choose? I tossed the ball back to
Rudy.

Chapter 25

BURN, BABY, BURN—OR NOT

℘

G*reg and I* decided to bring Charley to my appointment with the radiation oncologist. She'd seen me going to treatment after treatment and was always curious. She'd ask, "What did they do to you today, Mommy?" "What does the medicine look like?" and constantly "Why does it take so long?" I didn't always have answers for her—I was trying to be honest yet shelter her at the same time. I was relieved that she never questioned the validity of what I said. I think she just wanted answers and was all right with the ones I provided.

Since my experience at the hair salon, buying a wig, I'd wanted Charley to be as involved in the process as possible. Even before that, I had thought I might take her with me to my chemotherapy sessions until I realized that the minimum age for visitors is eighteen—a limit I discovered exists for the safety of patients as well as visitors, since chemotherapy drugs are so toxic. And realistically, although Charley is well behaved, the last thing anyone would want is a three-year-old having a meltdown in the middle of an infusion.

Charley was super excited. She was always excited to tag along where I was going, and stopping at Tim Hortons on the way made it more exciting. I told her the appointment was to talk to a doctor about "medicine machines." When we got to the office, she couldn't wait to see what would happen. She had a hard time sitting and couldn't stop asking questions: "Why do you have to get changed into something else?" "Why do you have to sit on that table?" "Why do Daddy and I have to sit on these chairs?" She especially wanted to know what was going to happen with the "medicine machine."

When Doctor 8 entered the room, he said hello to Greg and me, then turned to Charley, who immediately stopped fidgeting to focus all her attention on him. He crouched down to converse with her and asked how old she was, what her favorite color was, and what school she went to, and even talked about his own kids.

"Hey, Charley," he said after they had chatted for a while, "is it all right if I talk with your mom now and examine her?"

"What are you going to look at?"

"I'm going to check her all over to make sure she's healthy. Is that okay with you?" He gave me a questioning look, too, and I knew he wanted to make sure I was good with Charley's being there during my exam.

I nodded, and Charley said, "I'm good." She wasn't fazed at all by anything, and I figured that was because I'd been so careful to keep her in the loop right from the beginning. I lay back and Doctor 8 started feeling under my armpits and around the incision mark from my lumpectomy. I couldn't help but let out a little giggle, and Charley asked, "Does that tickle, Mommy?"

"It does." So much so that I had to hold it together to keep Doctor 8 from harm's way—my natural reaction was to swing at someone if they went near my armpits.

Greg and I were really impressed by Doctor 8. His gaining Charley's trust made all the difference in the world. She had no problem sitting and listening, and we were able to direct all of our attention to what he had to say without being distracted by a bored child. I was glad Charley felt so comfortable, because I was trying to hide my own unease. Would I have to have radiation on top of chemotherapy and surgery? What would radiation do to me? How long would a course of radiation be? If I didn't get it, would I have done everything possible to beat cancer?

But before I had a chance to even ask anything, Doctor 8 said, "I don't think radiation will be necessary. There are many reasons for that, but mainly it's based on your decision to have a double mastectomy." He explained that with a simple mastectomy (which I was having on the right breast), the entire breast tissue was removed, but the axillary lymph nodes remained. In a modified radical mastectomy (which I was having on the left breast), the entire breast tissue was removed, along with the axillary lymph nodes. "Because of all the tissue being removed, there will be nothing left to radiate."

I believed him right away. That might have seemed odd, but he'd won me over because of his talk with Charley—made me feel I could trust him. Even so, I had more questions. "What are the recurrence rates for the different procedures?"

"Four to 8 percent for lumpectomy and radiation over thirty years, and 1 to 2 percent for mastectomy."

"The lower the number, the better as far as I'm concerned—I say take my foot if you have to get the recurrence rate down." It sounded like I was joking, but I wasn't.

"Radiation would provide no further benefit. That is, of course, assuming that the results from the pathology are good."

"What exactly does that mean?"

"Good pathology means there's no cancer in any of the other lymph nodes taken out during your mastectomy, and that there's no other cancer in any tissue that's removed."

I sat back. My surgery was another month and a half away, and I would have to wait for pathology results after that. I realized I'd started chewing on my fingernails. Nothing would be certain until the results were in. I couldn't help but feel that I was stuck in time while everything around me kept happening. I'd had that feeling before when I was in a situation like this. My thoughts churned in my head, but I felt unable to process them. Charley behaved, thankfully, or perhaps I couldn't take in what was happening—Greg may have been talking with her or distracting her somehow—since my focus was all on every word coming out of Doctor 8's mouth. He stopped talking, and I sat there, stuck, until he started talking again.

"Because the tumor margins were clear when your surgeon performed the lumpectomy, only one of your lymph nodes was affected, and the cancer there was very small in size, it doesn't seem likely any more tissue would be affected. Those are also reasons why I don't think radiation will be necessary. On the off chance more cancer cells are found, we'll revisit the radiation discussion."

Doctor 8's reasoning was so logical, his manner so soothing, I felt myself relax somewhat.

"Which reconstruction surgeon are you going to?" he asked.

My thoughts coalesced, and I found I could speak. I told him.

"He does amazing work. You've got to see pictures."

"I can't wait to see." I chuckled unexpectedly. "Who would have ever thought that one day I'd be asking to see boob photos!" The mood in the room picked up.

"Can I come to the appointment to help you pick from the photos?" Greg asked jokingly.

"Not a chance!" I had to smile. Men! The size of my boobs was the least of my concerns. All I cared about was going to a surgeon who knew what he or she was doing, someone who would make me look and feel normal again.

Chapter 26

"REAL" OR FAKE?

$\mathcal{P}$

In the period between my appointment with the radiation oncologist and the appointment with the plastic surgeon, life remained very much the same. If my having almost no hair on my head, only a few measly eyelashes and eyebrows, and almost no hair on the rest of my body could be considered normal. And it was the dead of winter, too. What could be better?

I was getting tired of the no-hair thing (although I had to admit not shaving my legs was a blessing), but I was also getting used to it. I didn't care as much what people thought about how I looked, and I found it easier to get out of the house since the nausea had eased. There were rare glimpses of the sun, and whenever it was sunny, the kids and I would bundle up and get outside. The more I saw the sun, the more I looked ahead to spring, and I knew that by the time spring arrived, the chemotherapy part of my journey would be over.

I was looking forward to meeting my plastic surgeon, Doctor 9, to see those incredible boob photos. I asked Erin to join me for the appointment. I wanted her there for her opinion and to take notes. I also needed her along to watch Rudy. Charley was in day care that day, but I had no one else to take care of Rudy, so we bundled him up and tucked him into his car seat.

I'd done some research and knew going in to the appointment that there were likely two choices for reconstruction surgery: fake boobs made from silicone or saline, or boobs made from a part of my own body, most likely extra tissue from my stomach. While we were waiting in the doctor's reception area, I told Erin that I was worried about the fake boobs: that they could explode upon impact, and that my body could reject them. "With 'real' boobs, I'm pretty sure there won't be any rejection issues at all, and I'll get a tummy tuck at the same time."

"Bonus!" Erin said.

Doctor 9 walked in and I could tell Erin was as surprised as I was by how young and good-looking he was. His confident manner instantly made me feel comfortable. "I want to know everything that's going on with you," he said. "So why don't you tell me why you want to have reconstruction surgery?"

I gave him my history—the cancer, the lumpectomy, and the chemotherapy. Then he began explaining the two options for surgery—transabdominal reconstruction or expanders followed by implants. Rudy decided that would be the perfect time to poop. While Erin tended to him, I continued my conversation with Doctor 9 and was impressed by his focus. He wasn't fazed at all.

"The first step, by the surgical oncologist, would be to remove your breasts and most of the surrounding tissue, which extends up towards your collarbone and includes the lymph nodes on your left side," he said. "Your nipple would be removed first and tissue taken out through the hole where the nipple was. Then I'd cut two circular pieces of flesh the same size as your nipples out of your abdomen between your belly button and pubic bone. Those would fit right into the opening left by your old nipples." He looked at me to see if I was with him and drew a quick picture to show me what he meant.

I swallowed.

"In order to get the piece of flesh that will become your new breast in place, a portion of your ribs would be removed, then the flesh would be attached with microscopic blood vessels to keep it alive. All of that would take about six and a half to eight hours."

Erin looked at me, her eyebrows raised. I knew she was thinking the same thing I was: The surgery was so complicated. It was much more invasive than I'd realized. I was kind of freaking out.

"The recovery time would be five days in the hospital, then two to three months at home with no heavy lifting at all," Doctor 9 continued. "The benefit of this procedure is that it's a single operation. Once you recover from it, you're done. There will be no rejection issues and no need to come back to get filled up."

"What about the breasts ever leaking or exploding on impact?"

"No, no possibility of that. But because the breasts are formed using natural flesh, they could end up sagging just like regular breasts do over time, so they won't be permanently perky the way implants would be."

I was amazed at how naive I'd been. And what was the other procedure going to be like? I knew Erin was taking notes in between watching after Rudy, but there were more things I needed to know to make a decision. I tried to gather my thoughts. "What are the risks of this particular procedure?" I could hear my voice crack a little.

"Those microscopic blood vessels we use to attach the skin from your stomach can become pinched or twisted, and you could then lose that transplanted flesh. And hernias and scarring can form on your abdominal area."

He looked at my stomach.

"There *might* be enough tissue for me to do this procedure, but your breasts won't end up being extraordinarily large, I'm afraid."

He probably didn't realize, but he'd just paid me a compliment. I guess the Ab Ripper exercises were paying off. "That's okay, I never wanted large breasts in the first place, although I figured if I was going to go through all this surgery, I might as well come out with something substantial," I joked.

He smiled. I was glad I could manage to be funny under the circumstances.

"For implants, as with the other procedure, the surgical oncologist would remove your breast tissue up to your collarbone; however, I'd then remove most of the skin from the front of your breast, including your nipples. Since that's the case, you'd have expanders placed underneath your chest wall to stretch what's left of the remaining skin so I can place the implants where they need to go."

He showed me an example of an expander. They were like empty implants that had a little metal valve. "After your breasts are removed during surgery, the expanders would be filled with approximately 60 cubic centimeters—60 milliliters—of saline, and I'd stitch you up in a straight line horizontally on each breast. Starting four weeks after the surgery, you'd come in three or four times, depending on how big you want to go, each time two to three weeks apart, and I'll put a needle through your skin into the valves to fill each expander with around 100 cubic centimeters of saline."

"How will I know how large to go?"

"You live with the breasts after each fill and see how you like that size. Once you're comfortable with them as they are, we wait approximately six weeks. Then you come in for another surgery to remove the expanders and get implants to match the size."

"What are the implants made of?"

"A cohesive gel, similar to that of a gummy bear."

"And what are the risks?"

"Although it's less extensive and there are fewer possible complications, there is the chance that some years down the road you might need another surgery to get the implants repaired or replaced."

"What do you think, Erin?" I asked.

"The natural boobs made out of your tummy tissue are a way bigger procedure than I realized."

I could tell she was overwhelmed. I was, too, although I had gotten used to medical language being thrown at me.

Doctor 9 showed me an example of an implant, and Erin and I both felt it.

"You're right—it does feel like a gummy bear," I said. I tried to imagine what it would feel like inside me, and how it would feel to someone else.

He then opened up his computer and showed us photos upon photos of breasts.

"So you essentially created these?"

"Yes."

There was an entire section that didn't apply to me—breasts that had been augmented or reduced for cosmetic reasons. Then we looked at photos of breasts created from tummy tissue, and afterwards photos of breast reconstruction with implants. After looking at the photos I began to think I had a better idea which route I wanted to go, but I had to ask another question. "Which surgery do you think would be best for me?"

"I can't recommend one over another for you, given the circumstances," he said, but after a pause, he went on. "Because of your age and because of the great cosmetic effects we can get, as well as less operating time initially, I think the implant procedure would be the best option for you." That made me happy. If I was going to get new boobs, them being perky would be a bonus. And if I never had to wear a bra again, that would be even better.

"I went in thinking one thing," I said to Erin when we left. "Now I'm not positive. You know I've never been a big fan of fake boobs, because I always felt they looked so unnatural. After seeing those photos, though, I think the breast replacement implants look more natural than the breast augmentation implants. I don't want anything bigger, I just want something that looks like what was already there."

"There's so much to think about," Erin said. "I wouldn't know what to do."

"I do like that with implants I don't have to decide up front how big or small I want them to be."

"How perfect is that! You get to 'try them on' for size and see what works for you."

"True. But there's a lot on the downside." I appreciated that Erin was trying to be positive, but there was so much involved in both surgeries.

Once we got back to my place, Erin got Rudy out of his car seat and handed him to me. "He's getting hefty."

"Twenty-eight pounds now." I kissed Erin good-bye and shifted Rudy from one arm to the other to unlock the door. I had time to make a decision about the reconstruction, but regardless of which procedure I chose, there was one order of business I definitely needed to take care of. With my not being allowed any heavy lifting after either surgery, eleven-month-old Rudy would need to move from the comfort of his crib into a big-boy bed shortly after his first birthday on February 11. Even though I'd have some help, I couldn't ask someone to stay with me for a whole six weeks. While we had already babyproofed the kitchen, we desperately needed to baby-proof Rudy's bedroom. He'd taken ten steps the other day, all at once, and any day now would be walking everywhere, getting into everything. In fact, we'd nicknamed him Bamm-Bamm, he'd gotten so destructive.

It was the end of January, my mastectomy was scheduled for March 23, and we needed to begin Rudy's transition. Before that, though, I still had two more chemo treatments.

Chapter 27

OVERREACTION

❧

M*ary Kay, who* had sent me the *Believe* T-shirt I wore to the hair-shaving party, was due to arrive at my house and take me to my third Taxol treatment. I'll never forget our first conversation. She'd been the vice principal at my school when I was on maternity leave with Charley. Charley was having a hard time adjusting to day care and I couldn't stop stressing about that. I found myself in front of Mary Kay's office one day when I popped into the school, and I knocked on her door.

The next thing I knew, we ended up chatting for a good hour. I couldn't help but feel like I was in trouble at first, because Mary Kay looked at me so directly—and she was the vice principal!—but I desperately needed some distraction to keep myself from thinking about poor Charley, and Mary Kay provided it. After that chat, I felt as though I'd known her forever. She was such an honest, genuine, sincere and generous person. I was so happy to have her with me for that chemo appointment.

When she arrived at our house, Charley ambushed her. The kids loved her. "Hey!" Mary Kay said, and gave me a big hug after managing to detach herself from Charley. "Your eyebrows and eyelashes are looking good!"

She'd been getting the "hair play-by-play," as I called it, but I'd begun to fall behind in my updates. "I thought by now they'd be totally gone, but there are a few stragglers, and at least there are still those few. I'm feeling better again, too. Finally some relief from the aches and pains."

I grabbed my snacks, we kissed the kids good-bye, and we headed to the hospital. While she'd heard about the usual round of blood work, weighing, and so on, Mary Kay was kind of wide-eyed about it all and wanted to know everything that was happening. She hadn't been to this type of appointment with anyone else before. When my number was called in the chemo suite, I went in and sat down on a stretcher.

"What's that?" Mary Kay asked when the nurse handed me some pre-meds.

"It's to help counteract allergic reactions. I already took a bunch last night and early this morning. It's unlikely anything's going to happen, since I've already gone through this twice, but can't hurt." I propped myself up on a couple of pillows so I could look at Mary Kay more comfortably while we talked, and the nurse started the saline drip, checked my vitals, and hooked up the Taxol drip. "Okay, you're good to go," she said. "I'll be back to check on you in a bit."

Mary Kay pulled a chair close, and we started talking about all the changes that happened since she'd left my school. Before we could get into the real nitty-gritty, though—two minutes at most since the IV had been started—I had to stop.

"Are you okay?" Mary Kay asked.

I looked at her. She shifted in and out of focus, but I could see she looked worried. "Can you get the nurses?" Before I could finish asking, she was out of her chair. My head was congested, my chest felt tight, and I felt dizzy.

The nurses were at my side within seconds.

"She looks like a ghost," I heard Mary Kay say.

"I'm going to throw up." It was all I could do to grab whatever was handed to me before I vomited up everything in my stomach, including all of the pre-meds I'd taken. What on earth was going on?

"Stop the IV and check her vitals," a nurse said.

Within minutes, the awful feelings began to subside.

"I don't understand," I said. "How can the Taxol be causing a reaction now? I've already had two successful treatments."

The nurses were stumped. "We're not sure what's going on," one said. "For a reaction to happen during the third infusion is rare. It's probably not the Taxol."

The other nurse chimed in. "Also, typical reactions involve shortness of breath, flushing of the face, fever and/or chills, or hives, not vomiting."

"Maybe it's the flu or something you ate. We'll talk to the oncologist and see what he thinks."

I lay back on the stretcher. "I thought I was going to get away with just the achiness," I said to Mary Kay. "Not so lucky."

One of the nurses returned. "We're going to start the saline drip again, especially since you vomited, okay?"

I nodded, and she set to work. I was surprised to find I hadn't been embarrassed to throw up in front of everyone. The nurses had closed the curtain around me to give me some privacy and while I appreciated the gesture, I really didn't care what anyone thought. The whole thing reminded me of that moment when you're giving birth and realize there's a room full of people looking at your crotch, and you're in so much pain that at that moment that's the least of your worries.

The nurse finished, but I had to ask, "Did you start the Taxol drip?" I'd begun to experience the same sensations as before, although at least this time I didn't vomit.

I could tell from her expression that she had. "I'll stop it right away." She was puzzled. "Because all your symptoms are so atypical, we think your reaction is just coincidental. But to be on the safe side, we're going to give you more steroids and some Zofran for the nausea."

So I popped more pills, and after a half hour, when the drugs were well into my system, the Taxol drip was started again, slowly. I warily watched the drug dripping through the tube, waiting for something to happen, and a nurse stayed to watch over me. But nothing. After twenty minutes, the nurse stood up. "Great! No glitches. I'll be sure to make notes on your chart for next time." The rest of the infusion went uneventfully. When all of the Taxol was in my system, the monitor started beeping and the nurse returned to gently pull the IV line out of my hand and bandage me up.

"How are you feeling?" she asked. "Okay?"

"I think I'm good now." I picked up my coat and purse. "Thanks for bringing me," I said to Mary Kay.

"I'm glad I was able to be here with you for it," she said and squeezed my good hand.

We ventured down the hall to get my pre-meds for next time, and then to the elevators, grabbing a coffee in the lobby for the drive home. On the way, Mary Kay kept asking me how I was feeling, but I was fine—no more weird reactions. And luckily no more nausea.

Back at the house, Mary Kay walked me in and gave me a huge hug. "That was an experience."

If only she knew everything I'd been through.

⌀

"Mommy!" Charley jumped in my arms when she saw me.

The great thing about kids is that no matter how "abnormal" their parents' lives become, in kids' eyes, things keep going on as usual. I was bald, I was about to lose my boobs, and every other week I was being pumped full of some toxic chemicals, but the kids' lives didn't change much. Charley still went to day care a couple of days a week; we still went skating at the public ice rink just down the road, built castles and played princess and zoomed toy dump trucks around the house. Everything for them was normal, and it was important to me to keep it that way.

Having Rudy and Charley helped me keep my focus away from my treatments, away from my aches and pains, away from the baldness. Rudy, who had been only seven months old when I was diagnosed, would soon be turning one. He was walking everywhere and loved taking things from where they belonged and putting them in different places, and it still drove me nuts. I was thankful, though—it kept me busy, which was perfect.

He didn't have a clue what was going on, though, but Charley was becoming more attentive at times. She always wanted to rub my bald head, and cuddle with me when I was tired, too. On the odd occasion when I was able to sleep in, she'd come into my room, pull the blanket up around me and give me the gentlest kisses she's ever given. "I'm just coming in to check on you, Mama," she'd say.

She was incredibly perceptive about the chemo jargon we used, and although she didn't understand everything, she'd use the words fairly accurately. On one occasion, she bumped into my arm. "I'm sorry," she said. "I hope I didn't hurt you where you get your chemo."

"Oh, sweetie, no, you didn't!"

She was amazing, and without her energy and kisses my chemo days would have been much tougher. She was so excited for her birthday in March not only because she'd get presents but because I had told her back when I was beginning chemo that hopefully by her birthday my hair would start growing back. She'd remembered that and had been reminding me about it, so I'd been praying to the hair gods that it would happen.

I had only one more chemo treatment to go, and it was wonderful to think about how life would start getting back to normal. My kids were my world, and my desire to kick cancer in the butt grew stronger and stronger, because every day I had with them wasn't enough—I wanted more days. Many, many more.

Chapter 28

PLANNING AHEAD

N*ot only were* my kids amazing, my family was rock solid when it came to supporting me. My mother was always ready and willing to drop anything to be there for me and the kids, and Greg was, too. My sister was also always on hand to come to appointments with me, help with the kids, and she even came to massage my legs when they were feeling extra achy from the Taxol (she is a registered massage therapist). My brother, Braden, lives in Winnipeg, and while I knew how hard it was for him to be so far away from me while all this was going on, I knew he wanted to protect me and would have been there if he could.

They were all amazing. Then my grandmother fell ill.

"She has C. difficile," my mother said.

"What's that? How did she get it?" I asked.

"After a visit to the hospital. Apparently it's a bacterium that upsets the balance of healthy bacteria in the digestive system. People can die from it." It seemed that for the last month Grandma hadn't been eating well or drinking enough, and had lost twenty pounds. She had to be admitted to the hospital. I couldn't believe it. I felt terrible for my grandmother and my mother. My grandfather had passed away when I was four years old, and by the time I was thirty-three, my grandmother had already been living alone for almost thirty years. I couldn't even begin to imagine how tough that was. Now she was really sick, and my mother was feeling torn and stretched in every direction, dealing with her and me.

"I'm so sorry, Mom." When I found out what was going on, I was amazed that she hadn't already broken down. My mom worked as a seamstress for a local company, and while the owner was an extremely compassionate woman who was good to her and had told her she could take as much time off as she needed to be with me, things still must have been stressful.

"We'll get through it. Your grandmother is strong. She'll get out of the hospital and go home. You'll see. And we'll help her. All of us." Mom took me by the chin. "Don't worry. You don't have to do anything. Just pray for her, and I'll take care of everything."

I couldn't help but wonder how.

*

"Alana, I think we should just go ahead and build the house now," Greg said to me one night at the dinner table.

"I'm not sure that's a good idea." I was truly leery about doing anything while there was so much going on. "I don't know where this is going to take me."

"You're going to live another seventy years," Greg said. "We should build our dream home now so we'll have seventy years to live in it together."

I was nervous. We had planned to wait about five years to build on our piece of property—not that far off, but still a few years away. But I thought about my situation and about my grandmother's, and decided to take these examples to heart. We were learning from this experience, and I realized that I couldn't help but agree with Greg. I hugged him. "So what do we have to do?"

"Start thinking about how to make this house sellable."

I jumped in. "Start finalizing the house plans." The idea of that made me excited—we could make it exactly what we wanted.

"And look for builders," Greg added, ever practical. "We could move into a rental in the spring and start building in the summer."

"Somewhere in Crystal Beach. It would be great for the kids. We could go swimming every day, when we're not working on the house."

Something to look forward to for once! I smiled. Things were looking up.

Chapter 29

MISSION ACCOMPLISHED

February 22, the day of my last chemo session, arrived and I was happy—I was ending one phase and beginning another—although I underestimated how big a deal the event was for everyone.

"When a doctor gives you a prescription for antibiotics, you take them. When you're told you need to have a filling, you get it done," I said to my mom while I waited impatiently for Erin to pick me up.

"But this is a big thing, Alana."

"None of those things, or chemotherapy, seems like a big achievement to me." For me, it was a necessary journey, and even though it was difficult at times, it didn't seem like a great accomplishment.

Erin's thinking was more aligned with my mother's. She had her arms full when she arrived. "I baked you cupcakes to mark the occasion!" She was smiling so hard she looked like a little kid. Pink balloons bobbed in the air behind her, the ribbons wrapped around her fingers. "Look! The cupcakes have breasts and pink ribbons and flowers."

"They even have nipples!"

"I brought enough for all of you, and the chemo nurses and oncologists, too. I even made them vegan, so you can eat them." Then she pulled out what she'd been trying to hide, a large bristol board sign made by my niece and nephew. It read: *I Did It!*

"That's so amazing!" I hugged her.

The balloons, the sign, the cupcakes—everything made me realize that what my mom had said was true: What I'd undergone wasn't as minor as a prescription or a filling. Physically getting through the chemotherapy was rough—in fact, it was horrible. It was a huge accomplishment. I asked myself, Would I do it again? And the answer was a resounding *yes*! If it meant I could live for many, many more years, yes, I would do it as many times as necessary.

> I asked myself, Would I do it again? And the answer was a resounding yes! If it meant I could live for many, many more years, yes, I would do it as many times as necessary.

∽

The oncology appointment before my last chemo session was different from all the others. We discussed things we never had before, like my hair growth and my period. Talking about my hair coming back felt like a new beginning.

"You should have about half an inch to one inch of hair in about three months," Doctor 7 said. "So it will probably be that long before you feel comfortable going out in public without a hat."

"Charley is going to be thrilled," I said to Erin. "I promised her I'd have enough hair to put in a barrette by her birthday in March. By those calculations I should be right on target," I said with a grin. I turned my attention back to Doctor 7. "I haven't had my period since my first treatment and I'm having hot flashes. I know that's one of the potential side effects, I just don't know for how long."

"That happens. I'm afraid you might never have your period again."

I could tell Doctor 7 thought I'd be upset, but I honestly thought that was kind of a gift, although the hot flashes were driving me crazy.

"About 40 percent of women stay in menopause, but that depends how far they are from entering it in the first place. In any case, it will be at least a year or two before you get your period back, if that happens at all."

"And what about monitoring for recurrences of cancer?"

"We'll see you quite frequently—you'll come back for checkups in three months, six months, nine months, and so on."

"And you'll do blood work?"

"No. We'll look for any symptoms and do a physical exam."

That caught me off guard. I thought they'd monitor my blood work. "What about mammograms or MRIs?"

"Not unless you have symptoms again—aches or pains that aren't explainable."

I couldn't quite believe that that was all that would be done, but what could I say? I thanked her and we left for the chemo suite.

$\mathcal{P}$

"Cupcakes!" Everyone in the suite gathered around, oohing and aahing at Erin's baking skills.

I started to tear up. The chemo treatments sucked, but I'd enjoyed the presence of so many of my close friends and family along for the journey—having their company, but also discovering what they thought about the whole experience.

Greg was probably the one who was the most fascinated by the medical stuff. My mom was probably the most emotional, because I was her daughter, after all. I knew she would have traded places with me in a heartbeat if she could have. Melanie definitely brought the best snacks, and she made me laugh—oh, how she made me laugh! Nina was so kind, and because of her uncle, she knew exactly what to expect and what to say. Mary Kay was curious but also genuinely concerned, wanting to know everything she could to help. My brother-in-law, Doug, was great to have along because that gave us a chance to spend more time together than we ever had before and to get to know each other. And Erin: her big-breasted cupcakes and balloons probably made me more emotional than I had ever been on the entire journey so far.

Thinking about Erin made me think about Braden and his family. I think my having cancer was harder on Braden than I'd initially thought, simply because he was so far away. If he had been here, I knew he would have dropped everything to help me, no questions asked.

I lay back on the stretcher. My last infusion was going off without a hitch so far—no reaction or nausea, although I was exhausted. "Even though I know I'll be hurting again in a few days, this time it'll be different," I said to Erin. "When the aches and pains are gone, that's it." Next thing I knew, I felt something tapping me on my shoulder. It was the nurse. I had fallen asleep. The infusion was done. I was finished with chemotherapy.

"It seems surreal," I said to Erin.

We had the nurse take a picture of me with Erin's balloons and the *I Did It!* sign, as well as the few cupcakes that were left. I looked around for a minute. I was done with this room. I wouldn't see these people, these nurses anymore. Although I'd grown to love the chemo nurses, it was great knowing that I was leaving. Surgery was next in line. Then all I could do to help prevent a recurrence was exercise, eat well, take my vitamins and supplements, and enjoy life.

I couldn't help but feel a little shocked at that.

Part Five

TURNING THE CORNER

Chapter 30

THE NEW, BOOBLESS ME

"They *want to* move Grandma into a nursing home," my mom said. "She's not ready for that." Grandma had been in the hospital for about two weeks. Mom was devastated, and I was floored. I wasn't trying to be selfish, but I couldn't help but feel that everything in my life was one step forward, ten steps back. Why couldn't I catch a break? Why couldn't Grandma?

The nursing home wasn't far from where Grandma lived, but it wouldn't be the same as being at home. The nurses wouldn't have the same compassion as my mom or anyone else, because she wasn't *their* grandmother or *their* mother.

I took a deep breath. I tried to focus on the bright side. That wasn't always easy, but it was all I had. *Twenty-nine days until new boobs*, I thought. What can I do to get myself ready? There wasn't much, I realized, but what there was to do, I did. I tried to get my body into the best shape possible so it could physically endure another surgery. I drank smoothies, got lots of rest, and took the kids for a walk every day. About two weeks after chemo ended, I had another unwelcome surprise: My period was back. It had been nice not having it for four months. On the bright side of things, though—*Always look on the bright side!* I thought, somewhat bitterly—the hot flashes subsided. I renewed my supply of tampons.

Although most people would probably be nervous about getting their breasts cut off, I wasn't. For me, it was the easiest choice of all. And since my last surgery—to remove the cancerous lump—had been only five months earlier, I wasn't even apprehensive about being operated on the way I had been then. I wasn't concerned about the pain I'd feel afterwards, either. The idea of beginning this next leg of the journey was welcome—the coming pain was simply part of that.

I wasn't even sad about the fact that my own breasts—the ones that had fed my babies, the ones that were a part of me—would be gone. I had chosen to have a double mastectomy, and I decided I'd be excited about this, not sad. And since having them removed would give me a better survival rate, I was even glad to see them go. They had betrayed me, and I didn't want them to be a part of me anymore. I wasn't thinking that I was losing my breasts, but rather that I was ditching the ones that had turned on me. They were just skin; I would still have my life. And instead I would get a perky new set that most women would pay thousands of dollars for. It was a win-win situation, wasn't it?

&

When my alarm went off, I knew something was wrong.

"Greg, wake up." Everything sounded muffled.

"What is it?" he mumbled.

I went to the window and drew back the curtains. "There are huge drifts of snow everywhere."

He rolled out of bed. "Good thing we planned to leave early."

The surgery wasn't until nine A.M. I had to check in two hours before, and the drive from door to door under perfect conditions was an hour, so we wanted to leave at five-fifteen. We hadn't accounted for weather like this, though. "I'm glad Mom came over last night, or she would have gotten stuck in this. And I've already packed my bags." In my mind I was running through everything that needed to be done and I turned on the radio as we hurriedly dressed. Weather reports were warning that one of the worst snowstorms of the year was rocking our region. We raced out to the kitchen, and Mom came in as we ran around, Greg grabbing a bite and me making sure everything was set for the kids while I'd be away.

"Do you have everything, Alana?" she asked sleepily.

"I'm good, Mom. Thanks. The kids' snowsuits are in the front closet, okay?"

"Why are you in such a rush?"

"The weather is terrible, Mom. We have to go." And with that, we dashed out.

We were on the roads before any plows, salt trucks or other cars, and were essentially clearing a path for everyone else. We both had never seen anything like it before. The major highways were covered with at least six inches of snow, and the visibility was so minimal we weren't sure where the road began or ended. Eventually, more people joined us, but many of them passed us and ended up swerving out of control. We saw at least eight cars in the ditches and had to stop for a full twenty minutes for one accident. My knuckles were white, and I wasn't even driving. I kept saying to myself over and over again, "Please, just get me there." I didn't want to miss the surgery.

At almost seven A.M., exactly when we should have been checking in, we were twenty minutes away. I called the hospital. "I'm on my way," I said. "Don't start without me."

Greg began laughing, and I joined in. We were both so nervous. I couldn't believe I'd said that.

Finally we arrived. Greg pulled up to the main entrance to let me out, and I had the door open almost before he stopped. I ran in to register while he parked. My heart was pounding from the race to the admissions office, but I had made it. I was ushered in to the prep room. This time I knew the routine—gown, bootees, IV, shot of heparin. It was like an assembly line— there were eight operating rooms and eight patients being prepped at the same time—and it was all ticking along like clockwork despite the blizzard. By the time I was done, Greg appeared. Five minutes before my surgery I was escorted from the prep area to the operating room.

"Call Mom, please, to let her know we made it and that I'm on my way in."

"I will. Are you ready?"

"Ready as I'll ever be. See you in a bit," I said, and headed off to the operating room. I was definitely not as scared as the first time. In fact, I felt like a bit of a pro as I walked in, excited, confident, as if there was a big weight about to be removed from my shoulders—in this case, though, the weight was literal. After I sat down on the operating table, the head nurse introduced me to the other nurses, then asked me to describe in my own words the procedure that was being done. "That way we're sure we're all on the same page," she said.

"I'm having a bilateral mastectomy with expanders put in, and all of the lymph nodes under my left armpit removed."

"Perfect. Can you lie down, please."

I did, my arms were strapped to the table, and the anesthesiologist began the gas.

"Please count backwards."

"Five, four, three, two . . ."

✑

I woke up in the recovery room at 11:20 A.M. I looked for Greg, but couldn't see him anywhere. I felt a lot of pressure on my chest.

A nurse noticed I was awake. "How are you doing?" she asked.

"Groggy. Much groggier than after my last surgery."

"Have some water. It'll make you feel better."

I did, then fell back asleep again. I woke up when I felt myself being moved. I was on a stretcher being rolled through the hallways, into an elevator, down a hall, and into a private room. I was groggy and the pain was beginning to creep up on me, especially since I was being moved. I asked the orderly the time. It was 12:30. Greg showed up a short time later, around 12:45.

"How are you?" He kissed me.

"I need some painkillers," I croaked. The pain was starting to come on hard and fast. The effects of the anesthetic had lasted what seemed a long time, but were wearing off by then. "I feel as though there are elephants sitting on my chest, and they keep getting heavier and heavier."

"I'll get a nurse."

I tried not to think of the pain while Greg was gone. I tried not to think of anything. Fifteen minutes later, which seemed like an eternity, the nurse arrived with morphine. Thankfully it came in an IV bag—that meant it could be added into my IV, which was already in place and wouldn't take too long to kick in. I was desperate. I watched her hook up the bag and attach the tube to my IV line. I couldn't wait for the morphine to start dripping into me, for the awful feeling to fade away.

"We were wondering if I would be able to stay?" Greg asked the nurse.

"We don't usually let people stay overnight."

"Since the weather is so bad, and the roads are terrible, we were hoping you might make an exception."

I crossed my fingers. I didn't want to be left alone, and I knew I'd need help, someone to fetch me medicine and help me go to the washroom. I felt overwhelmed and emotionally stunned. I didn't want to talk, partly because I was groggy, but more because I had just had two body parts removed. I was afraid to touch myself, afraid to see what I looked like, yet relieved at

the same time that I no longer needed to worry. After just a bit of convincing, she gave in. She even brought Greg a cot to sleep on.

Once I started moving about, I realized just how limited my movement
would be and how incredibly sore I was. Even worse, I suddenly became
aware of the effects of the IV fluid. "I need to go pee," I said to Greg. I
hadn't drunk much, but I'd gone through a few saline bags already that I
knew of. "Can you please help me get up?"

"Sure. What do you need?" Greg asked, uncertain what exactly to do.

"Everything," I said. I was embarrassed. "Getting up off the bed seems
impossible." I couldn't figure out what to do; it was so awkward—I had to
bring the IV stand with me, since I was hooked up to it. "Pushing myself
up off the bed is so unbelievably painful. I never realized how many muscles
in my chest I use to do that."

Slowly but surely, Greg adjusted the bed so that it was as upright as it
could possibly be. Where were the nurses when I needed them? With my
one hand on the bed and the other on the IV pole, and Greg's hand ready to
catch me but not sure where to hold on to me, I awkwardly and cautiously
inched my way off the bed and shuffled to the bathroom. When I managed to sit down and pee, it felt like the longest pee ever. I started laughing
in amazement, but caught myself right away because that hurt. I finished,
covered myself up and shuffled back to my bed. The whole process took
about twenty minutes.

"I'm glad they let me stay," Greg said.

"Fortunately I can wipe myself, because I swear if I couldn't do that, I
might honestly start crying." He propped me up and tucked pillows where I
needed them. He was a huge help all night. It was unfathomable to me how
I would have coped without his help. He put my slippers on, took them off,
gave me water, and did everything else I needed and that we'd taken for
granted I'd be able to do. The morphine helped, but not enough. I hurt like
hell. If I was registering my pain on a scale of ten, it dropped it only from
a nine to about a seven.

"I'm afraid you can only get it every four hours," the nurse said.

"But it's wearing off after three."

"I'm sorry, but I can't increase the frequency."

The only other time I had received morphine was during childbirth, when it had seemed to work. "Makes me realize how excruciating this pain is," I told Greg. Sleeping was difficult. I was used to lying on my side and stomach, and couldn't do that. Lying on my back all night long was awful.

With morning came a new nurse and another round of morphine. "How are you doing?"

"Not good. It hurts."

"You should be feeling better with the morphine. Why don't we try some Percocet?"

"Anything to help." I forgot my earlier reservations about the drug.

"It'll make you more drowsy than the morphine," she warned, "but less constipated, if that's been a problem." I hadn't noticed an issue because I hadn't eaten much since the surgery, but that was certainly something I wanted to avoid. And drowsiness wasn't a negative. Percocet it was! Within about twenty minutes of swallowing that magical pill, I realized it would be my drug of choice—it dropped the pain to a five and relaxed me. I closed my eyes and dropped off for about an hour, oblivious to what was going on around me. When I woke up, around eight A.M., I was feeling a bit better. I knew the more I slept, the less I would hurt. And as I began to feel better, I was anxious to get through the snowstorm and back home.

"You'll need to have a quick visit from the surgeons first, and then the doctor on call has to discharge you," the nurse said when she came back. "And I also need to show you how to take care of the drains that have been inserted. Let's do that now before the doctor comes." Before I had a chance to argue, she propped me up and started undressing my wounds.

I had to face my new boobless body, whether I liked it or not. I wasn't looking forward to that. I looked down. I still had my gown on, but I noticed a definite change. I wasn't as flat-chested as I had imagined I would be. In fact, I was happily surprised at the size of the breasts I already had. There were also three drains—one on my right side and two on my left. They were long tubes, and at the end of each was a clear plastic bottle or reservoir, about the size of those plastic lemons filled with lemon juice that you can buy at the grocery store. I felt like Frankenstein's monster.

"The reservoir has a clip so you can attach it to your clothing." The nurse showed me what she meant. "That way it won't continually pull away from the incision site." On the inside of my body, underneath my new implants, she explained, there was a flat piece of plastic that had a bunch of holes in it to help with drainage. "The drains need to be 'milked' regularly because they act like a siphon system. You have to squeeze all the air out of the bottle to create suction. That will drain excess fluid from the surgery site."

I'm positive both Greg and I looked appalled and fascinated at the same time.

"And just pull the tubing, which is stretchy, gently a few times to force any fluid that's in it to the end of the tube, where it'll collect in this reservoir." The reservoir was clear. She showed us the volume measurements that were marked on the side. "Measure the fluid, then record the volume, and each time you do that, empty and reattach the reservoir. You'll need to do that once every three to four hours at first for each drain. As time goes on, the reservoirs will collect less and less fluid and you'll need to empty them less frequently."

"When can the drains come out?"

"When you collect less than 25 milliliters in a day. A home-care nurse will come and remove them. If at any point you begin bleeding from the incisions, the reservoirs collect blood, or the fluid isn't becoming increasingly clear as time progresses, go to the emergency room right away."

Yikes! I thought. But I assured her I understood everything, and she left. "Everything always seems so complicated," I said to Greg, "but I know I'll get the hang of it."

Despite my desire to get away, it wasn't until just before lunchtime that both my surgical oncologist, Doctor 7, and plastic surgeon, Doctor 9, came to check me out. "The wounds look good," Doctor 7 said as she peered at my chest. "They should heal nicely. And although I can't be 100 percent sure until the pathology results come in, I'm fairly confident your lymph nodes were clear when I removed them, which would mean the cancer didn't spread anywhere other than your breast tissue."

Greg squeezed my hand.

"I'm also fairly confident I removed all of the cancerous tissue, but again I can't be 100 percent positive until the results come back, which should be in a few weeks."

Waiting. Always waiting. I looked at Doctor 7. Even though what she'd said wasn't a guarantee, I was going to trust her. I had to be able to move forward. For my own sanity.

Doctor 9 asked how I was feeling.

"Better now that I've taken Percocet. I felt a lot of pressure on my chest and the morphine wasn't working."

He nodded. "That's understandable. When I put expanders in, they're each usually filled with 60 cubic centimeters of saline. I felt you'd be able to handle more, so I put 120 cubic centimeters in."

"Oh?" That explained how I was feeling! "Why did you feel I could handle it?" I asked, because it honestly didn't feel that way. I laughed as I said it, because I didn't want to seem rude but wished I hadn't—I'd forgotten laughing hurt.

"You're young and healthy, which means your skin is more elastic and will be able to adjust rapidly to the change."

I tried to look at it optimistically: this meant I would leave the hospital not as flat-chested and would have fewer subsequent appointments for "fill-ups." It also explained why when I looked down for the first time I had bigger "mounds" than I initially thought I would. The two surgeons left, and I was just about to say to Greg, "I wonder how long it will take before we get out of here," when the doctor on call showed up. I hadn't seen him before, but I didn't care. I just wanted to be on our way home, with my new set of breasts.

"How are you feeling?" he asked, and looked at my chart.

"Like I'm ready to go home."

He smiled. "I'm going to check your incisions, and if they're healing nicely, I'll discharge you." He undid my bandages ever so gently, and while he looked down, I looked straight ahead—I wasn't ready to look again. "The surgeon did a nice job. These are going to heal nicely." I was happy to take his word for it and also to hear him sounding so impressed. He signed papers in my chart. "You're free to go."

I would have jumped out of the bed if I could have. As it was, I carefully shifted myself out and Greg helped me get into the wheelchair an orderly had brought into the room earlier. As he'd done on our last trip out of the hospital, Greg wheeled me to the front door of the hospital, but once again I then walked to the car. I was determined to do this, although I was a lot slower than the last time. I stole a pillow from the hospital and placed it between my chest and the seat belt. I couldn't bear the thought of the seat belt rubbing against me, nor did I want it to disrupt any of the stitches. I leaned the seat back and dozed off on the way home. Before I knew it, we were pulling in the driveway.

"Hey, Mom," I said as I walked into the kitchen. She was making snacks for the kids, who were in the living room. I peeked around the corner; they were building block towers. They saw me and raced over. I dropped onto a kitchen chair—I didn't want to be bumped into or knocked over—and braced myself for a big hug.

"We missed you, Mommy," Charley shouted, and started crawling onto my lap.

"Charley, be careful!" my mom said and tried to pull her off me. "You're going to hurt her."

"It's okay, Mom. Charley, come sit beside me on the couch," I said, getting up slowly. Mom finished getting the snacks together and brought them into the living room. I knew she was trying to distract the kids so they wouldn't be all over me, and I gave her a grateful glance.

Mom took care of everything to do with the kids for the next few days, so I could just hang out with them. She forced me to nap, which helped the healing process, and reminded me to do the stretches recommended by the doctors to maintain the range of motion in my arms, since the surgery would affect that.

She also reminded me to empty the drains. They were proving to be annoying—it was a pain to milk the tubing, empty the reservoirs, then clip them back on again—yet it was also fascinating to have three long tubes sticking out of my body and draining fluid. Gross, too. The fluid was at first red, then pink, yellow and almost clear, a transformation that was a sign things were going well. There was an average of 40 to 50 milliliters per day for the first two days, then 20 to 30 milliliters for the next couple of days. I had to wait till that amount was consistently down to less than 25 milliliters during a twenty-four-hour period for the drains to be removed, although both drains on my left side had to be removed on separate days. I could not wait for all of them to be gone.

Chapter 31

SIGNS OF EMOTION

✌

I hadn't been able to shower in six full days; cautious baths were all I could manage.

"How do you do it?" Melanie asked one day when we were chatting on the phone.

"I sit on the side of the tub, put the reservoir bottles on the ledge beside me, then carefully slip into the water. I just have to watch that I don't get the drains and everything wet."

"What a pain!"

"Surprisingly, it's not that bad compared to feeling sick." That was true. The drains were gross, yes; a bit awkward—they'd pinch at times under my ribs or in my side where they poked out of my body, depending on how I moved—but particularly inconvenient, no. And I'd take them over constant nausea. But when the fluids decreased enough that it was time for the home-care nurse to come and remove them, I had to admit I was pretty happy.

When the nurse arrived, Greg and I led her into our bedroom. I lay down on my side, as instructed, and she explained what was going to happen while she prepped her supplies.

"I'll take out the stitch that's holding the drain in, then count down from three. When I get to zero, it'll be over."

"That's it?" Greg said.

"That's it. And within an hour, the holes will be completely closed up."

I looked back at her; she was standing behind me, so she'd be able to get a better grip on the drains, I guessed. How could it possibly be that easy?

She took hold of the tube, began counting, and said, "Take a deep breath!" and pulled till the whole drain came free. Greg, who was standing beside the nurse so he could watch, gasped in shock, I presume. I started laughing at his reaction; I was amazed it didn't hurt. I wondered if that was because I was numb from the surgery.

"I can't believe how long it is," Greg said. I could hear the awe in his voice. "Do you want to see it, Alana?"

"No," I said, almost before he finished asking. I was staring out the window, and I refused to shift my focus. I was sure we'd been told the drains were 8 centimeters long, but from the sound of Greg's voice, I couldn't help but think they were much longer. After the nurse removed the second one, he showed it to me. It was huge! In fact, each drain was 8 *inches* long—so long they must have been crossing over each other inside of me.

The nurse packed up. "I'll be back tomorrow to take out that third drain." I glanced at my watch; by the time she left, only fifteen minutes had gone by.

The next day Greg took the drains to work; the nurse had left them behind. When he got home he was buzzing. "You should have seen the guys' faces. They turned green. They couldn't believe you had those in your body."

Later that night I was the one who was uncomfortable.

"What's wrong?" Greg asked, as he noticed me shifting in bed.

"I can't lie on my stomach like I used to, I can't lie on my sides because I feel pressure, and I'm completely not used to sleeping on my back." I thought back to that night in the hospital after I'd had the breast-reconstruction surgery and how awful that had been. Percocet wasn't an option anymore, though, because I'd completely finished my prescription and had nothing left. I was frustrated and getting myself wound up.

"Just try to relax," Greg said.

I couldn't at that moment. I felt mangled and alone. Each time the painkillers started wearing off, I'd realize how I actually felt. The pain wasn't so much a stabbing or piercing feeling, but rather an incredibly uncomfortable feeling of pressure, as if I had something pushing against my rib cage—not surprising considering the things inside me were called "expanders." Although the pain was more intense than it would have been had the doctor not put extra saline into the expanders right away, I was happy he'd made that decision because I was now one step closer to the end result. I could live with the pain. I could. At least that's what I kept telling myself. Then the painkillers would wear off again.

I couldn't sleep, I hurt so much, and I couldn't stop thinking. I didn't have the slightest desire to see my new breasts—or lack thereof. Bandages concealed most of my chest. On top of the bandages I wore a wrap that looked like a tube top to hold everything in place. The tube top seemed like a neat idea until I found out what it actually was: a pair of hospital-supplied underwear with the crotch cut out. Finally morning came. I must have fallen asleep at some point, and that must have done me some good, since I didn't feel as helpless as I did the night before. But the idea that a part of my body had just been removed was haunting me.

"What's the matter?" Mom said when I joined her in the kitchen for a coffee.

"It's weird." I shrugged, hesitating. "I'm glad they're gone, because I'm glad that I don't have to deal with it anymore, but I literally just had my boobs chopped off. That's hard to get used to."

She hugged me. "I can't say it's okay. And I can't say I understand, because I don't. It is what it is, and it's something you had to do, and you are stronger because of it."

"Thanks, Mom. You're right. As usual." I took a big swallow of coffee and the two of us sat there, silent at the kitchen table.

The pain got more bearable over the next few days. As that happened, I started to feel more curious. I had tried not to look at myself when the home-care nurse had changed the bandages—I wasn't ready for that yet—but I couldn't avoid glimpses. When she stopped coming, I was on my own, though, and I decided it was time to have a good look.

I shut myself in the bathroom off the master bedroom. Charley was less likely to come looking for me there. I stared at myself in the mirror and steeled myself for the first glimpse of the new me. It was some minutes before I could remove the tube top. I took a deep breath, then removed the first layer of bandages. It was kind of like unwrapping one of those presents that someone has covered in layers of paper, and I didn't know when I was going to get to the bottom. There were a couple of layers of thick gauze to take off, and then a thinner piece of gauze that was stuck in a square patch over my breast. I slowly peeled that off, not wanting it to stick to anything or tear any stitches.

I shut myself in the bathroom off the master bedroom. . . . I stared at myself in the mirror and steeled myself for the first glimpse of the new me.

Then there it was, the last piece of medical tape that was covering my wound. Ever so gently, I began to remove the tape. When it came away from my skin, my two mastectomy scars were staring right at me.

The nipples were gone, which was weird to see, or not see, I had to admit. Two horizontal incisions ran across each side of my chest. They were impressive: The doctor had done an amazing job, and the stitches weren't at all visible on the outside. There was bruising—large blue and purple patches stretching from side to side. I couldn't figure out how much of the mounds I saw were as a result of swelling or my new breasts. I touched them tentatively. They were numb, somehow didn't feel a part of me. But I felt good about how great my new breasts looked. I wanted to show them off to other people.

I opened the door and called out to the living room.

"Greg, can you come here for a minute?"

He was there in seconds, thinking something was wrong.

"Do you want to see?" I asked, knowing already what the answer would be.

"Sure!" And without hesitation, I removed the tape that I had just put back on.

"Wow, it looks really good! I was expecting more stitches!"

"I know. Me too." I yelled out again. "Mom, come here!" Greg left to trade places with my mom so he could watch the kids.

"Do you want to see my scars?"

"Sure!"

I lifted the tape again.

She cringed, thinking that it hurt me, then smiled. "Wow, Alana, I'm impressed. I mean, I didn't know what to expect, but it's better than I expected."

We were all expecting scars like those on Frankenstein's monster, and that certainly wasn't the case. It looked like the skin had been folded over in such a way that the stitches were neatly tucked inside. It was beyond fascinating, and I was beyond thrilled.

A short while later, a friend of mine, Adel, popped by to drop off some homemade treats. I wanted to get her opinion, too. We went to the bathroom, and I pulled off my top and removed the bandages.

"Oh my god, Alana! They look amazing!" She almost started crying. "I thought it would be much worse. I thought there would be more scars or something—but not this."

"They're great, aren't they?" I couldn't stop smiling. "I didn't think they'd look this good at this point, either. And I have to admit no nipples isn't as bizarre as I thought it would be."

"How are you feeling otherwise?" she asked.

"I'm pretty happy," I said. Of course, if she'd asked me that morning, my answer would have been different. What a difference seeing the amazing work my plastic surgeon had done had made!

❧

I was determined to do my stretching exercises every day. The sooner I could move properly, the sooner I'd be able to do everything I used to. The exercises were to regain full range of movement. I'd been given a list for the first seven days after surgery, then more to do after that. For the most part, I had to stand near a wall and try to inch my arms up the wall. Luckily I was able to do the exercises while keeping an eye on the kids. But the stretches were difficult—I found it hard to move my arms to shoulder height and couldn't lift anything over five pounds.

"Don't overdo it," Mom said when she saw me wincing in pain.

"I need to get back to normal."

"You might end up worse if you push it too far."

I was impatient, though. In my mind I wasn't getting back to my "normal self" fast enough. I decided to go to physiotherapy. The sessions would be two times a week for four weeks. After a single session, I had already noticed a slight improvement—I could move a tiny bit farther. I was glad. Being dependent on other people all the time was driving me crazy. I hated it. Mom was staying with us for a few weeks, and family and friends had scheduled "helping" days—which was all wonderful in theory and in practice. Logically I knew that. Except I desperately wanted to get back into the swing of things.

"Just let us help," my mother kept saying.

"I feel as though I've already taken up so much of everyone's time. I don't want to bother anyone anymore."

"You're not supposed to do things. You might hurt yourself."

"I know, and I have to force myself not to, but I'm frustrated you're missing out on work because of me. I'm angry that Greg doesn't get paid sick days to stay home to help, and while I'm so grateful people are willing and able to drop everything they're doing to help me out, I wish they didn't have to."

"People want to help. Otherwise they feel helpless. Sometimes you just have to learn to say thank you."

Still, I couldn't help but think it was my responsibility to get better so we could all get back to normal. I tried to ask for just what I needed, but it felt as though everyone except my mom thought I was getting quite good at delegating. Greg even asked me at one point to be patient. I was hurt, I admit it. I wasn't trying to be demanding, but I also was unwillingly forced into the role of delegator instead of my old role of doer. And until my six weeks of recovery were up, I had no choice in the matter.

♎

When I was finally able to go see my grandmother, it had been a few weeks since she'd been diagnosed with C. difficile. I hadn't visited her in all that time, especially while she was in the hospital, because no one wanted me to take a chance of getting sick—that was a very real possibility. But now she was in a nursing home, and well enough that I could go visit her.

When I walked into her room, I was taken aback. This was not the grandmother I knew. I started crying and couldn't stop. I sobbed for a good twenty minutes. She looked sad, lonely, weak and frail, sitting in a chair in the corner of the room—but I realized that all of the emotion I had been bottling up inside for the last six months was now flooding out of me.

My poor grandmother! I felt bad that I just went there and cried, but I felt comfortable letting it all out with her, and I clearly needed that release. I know she understood. She told me I would be okay and consoled me, and we just sat there, two sick people together, holding hands, side by side. It was the kind of closeness I would always remember.

Chapter 32

ABIDING SCARS

*M*y *breasts were* healing nicely. The bruises were fading, the stitches dissolving, and the scabs falling off. I massaged and moisturized them daily to speed things along. I had nothing to compare them to, but as far as the scars were concerned, I thought my plastic surgeon had done a fantastic job and I was sure they would look great in the end. What I was going through was just a process. It was weird touching my breasts because I had no sensation in my chest. I could feel what I was doing in my hands, obviously, but not in my breasts. And they weren't smooth and round and supple anymore, either. They were firm, immovable, and a slightly odd shape because of the expanders. I could feel the seams of those near my chest wall. Nothing about them felt natural.

It was clear that my body had been through a battle. I had been wounded, scarred forever. I was trying not to let that change my life. In fact, in many ways the scars were the only reminder that cancer had wormed its way into my life. That and these new mounds, which were far from the little deflated saggy post-baby boobs that I had seen in the mirror every day.

I was anxious to move on. There were so many more physical procedures to come before the journey would officially be over, but I decided I would try to embrace my scars the same way that I had embraced the loss of my hair. They made me different. They were proof that I had kicked cancer's butt.

"Maybe it's a good thing we have scars," I said to my mother. "They show us and others what we've overcome. Remind us how strong we truly are. Tell our story."

> It was clear that my body had been through a battle. I had been wounded, scarred forever. I was trying not to let that change my life.

A couple of weeks after the surgery, my mom went back to work and I had to start fending for myself at home with the kids. I was so tired, though. Sleep was a chore. The expanders were hard, sticking out below my skin in some places, and it felt as though they moved around underneath my chest muscle, which was disconcerting. So I slept on my back without a pillow under my head, using one under my knees instead. I definitely didn't get a deep or restful sleep, and the days became unbearably long. Every once in a while I took an Ativan just so I could get a deep sleep and play catch-up.

I also had trouble sleeping because I was worried. "I can't stop thinking about the pathology results," I said to Greg.

"No matter how many times we've had to wait, it never gets easier, does it?"

"It doesn't. I can't stop thinking about the first 'fill-up' with the plastic surgeon, either. I can't help but wonder if it'll make everything hurt all over again."

There were days when I was home alone with Charley and Rudy that it seemed impossible for me to keep my eyes open, even as early as ten in the morning. One day I was sitting next to the couch while the kids were playing on the floor, and I'm sure I dozed off. I jerked awake suddenly and realized Rudy was up on the couch. I didn't even notice him crawling up there. *What kind of horrible mother am I?* I thought. I opened up some windows and made a coffee in an attempt to wake myself up.

I kept thinking back to when I was a new mom and everyone told me, "Sleep when the baby sleeps!" Like any new mother, though, I did the opposite. I used naptime to do laundry, wash dishes and clean the house. I learned from my mistakes, though, and started heeding that advice. We started a new afternoon ritual: When Rudy went down for a nap, Charley and I would lie down together on the couch. She'd chill out and watch a bit of television, and I could close my eyes for a few minutes. I didn't ever get a good sleep, but it was a necessity. I took every single opportunity to nap.

As I got more rest, things started to get better all around. My appetite began to come back, and my energy levels increased a little each day. The thing I was most thrilled about, though, was that my hair was starting to come in again. At first there was just the faintest peach fuzz. I wasn't even sure I was seeing what I thought I was.

"Greg, come look!"

"What?"

"There's more hair," I said. He thought I was crazy. I was constantly asking him to look to see if there was new hair growing in. But there was, and more on the top of my head than on the sides. "I feel like Mr. T!" I joked. "I'm definitely going to have to get a trim any day now to even things out." And my eyebrows and eyelashes were coming back, too. But while the doctors and nurses had all said my hair would grow in quickly, the process wasn't as quick as I wanted it to be.

One day Adriana called me from school. As she'd discovered more about the ordeal I was undergoing, Adriana became committed to the fight against breast cancer—more specifically "my breast cancer," as she called it. After all, she had been one of the founding members of the Boobie Brigade and also hadn't hesitated to join the Dinner Club. The fact that I was sick, that I had cancer, didn't scare her away at all, the way it did a lot of people. "I've become one of the organizers of Relay for Life, and I'm looking for team members."

"What is the relay, exactly?"

"I need to get together a team of ten people who'll take turns walking or running around a track to raise money for the Canadian Cancer Society. The event will take place at the high school in Niagara Falls. It goes on the whole night, and we can bring lots of food, a tent, and maybe even sneak in some wine! It'll be a fun night!"

"I'm in!" I was so excited.

"You don't even know the nitty-gritty yet." Adriana said. She was used to my exuberance. "I have to get pledges of at least $100 from each of the ten people I choose to be on my team. Our team needs to raise $1,000 all together."

"No worries!" That would be a piece of cake. I sat down and sent out an e-mail to everyone on my list of contacts.

Erin was the first to respond. "I'm in for $50."

People had been so amazingly supportive ever since I'd been diagnosed, I wasn't surprised when the donations started pouring in from there. It wasn't long before I reached the goal for my team—then surpassed it.

<p>

I continually told myself that the cancer was gone, but having that confirmed by the pathology results would mean I could rest easy. I was trying so hard not to think about the possibility that there was more cancer, but couldn't voice my concerns to anyone else. If there was cancer, that would mean radiation, possibly more surgery, even chemotherapy again. I wasn't prepared for that. I tried not to let those nasty thoughts sneak into my head, but it was so hard.

The night before my pathology appointment, I went to bed with the same thoughts I'd had before: *The news I'll get tomorrow—good or bad—will change my life.* When Greg's alarm went off in the morning, I was exhausted. I hadn't slept much. I went out to the kitchen to make coffee and grab a few minutes by myself to try to relax. It didn't help.

Greg got up and so did the kids. I needed to shower and get the kids ready to go. Rudy was at last old enough to go to day care, which was a relief.

"Try not to worry, Alana. I'm sure you'll be fine," Greg said as he left.

I got the kids bundled up and into the car. Luckily they were quiet on the way over to the day care, and Charley was good with the drop-off.

"I love you," I said to her as I gave her a big squeeze.

"I love you, too," she said, and went off to play with her little friends.

Rudy had a tough time letting go once in a while, and this was one of those days. Maybe he sensed that I was having a tough time, too. In any case, the day-care worker had to pry him from my arms.

"He'll be fine," she said. "Honestly, he usually stops crying before you even leave the building." While that might have been true, it just wasn't a good start to the day. I wiped a tear from my eye, got in the car and turned on the music to distract myself. I still had to pick my mother up. When she saw me, she knew.

"You're worried," she said.

"I wish we could get the results first," I said. "But my fill appointment is first."

We walked into admitting, and I started scrambling about in my purse.

"What's the matter?" Mom asked.

"I can't find my health card." I couldn't believe it. "What if they postpone or even cancel the fill?"

"I'm sure they won't."

I explained the situation to the nurse in admitting.

"Let me look you up." She typed away on her computer. "I found you. You can go ahead."

I was so relieved. We walked down the hallway to the outpatient wing. I wondered how my mother was going to handle the procedure. I didn't say anything to her about what was going to happen. I figured anticipation would make things worse.

Before the procedure I had to fill out paperwork at the main reception area. Then I was called into another room to go over my medical history with a nurse and have my blood pressure taken. After that we went back out to wait. There were about five other people waiting, too, and I wondered what they were all there for. "I wonder why mammograms and breast screening are supposed to be most important in women over fifty?" I said to my mother. "Look at everyone here. They're almost all younger, just like me." Maybe they weren't cancer survivors, though. Some of them may have been there for a good old plastic surgery enhancement. If so, I couldn't help but think, *I wish life were that easy.*

When my name was called, Mom and I went to an exam room, where a nurse left a gown with me and asked me to put it on, before she discreetly left. After a moment there was a knock on the door, and Doctor 9, my plastic surgeon, and the nurse who took my blood pressure came in.

"How are you, Alana? How are you feeling? Any pain or soreness?"

"I'm quite numb."

"That's not surprising. Why don't you lie down so I can examine you?"

He felt around the incision, around my chest wall where the seams of the expanders were, and in my armpit area. There was a little bit of swelling on my left side under my armpit where the drains had been removed.

"Is that normal?" I asked.

"Absolutely. It's just a bit of fluid left over from when the drains were in and should dissipate over time. I'm going to use a magnet to find the port in the expander." He marked the spot with a pen and filled a needle with saline. "I suggest we start with 60 cubic centimeters in each breast, bringing it up to 180 cubic centimeters, because we don't know how you'll feel after this."

"Sounds good to me," I said. I was amazed I could talk. The needle was the longest, thickest needle I had ever seen. He pushed it into my breast. Surprisingly, it didn't hurt at all. There was just some pressure.

He explained, "I'm moving this through the port and into the expander."

I looked away, staring into the nurse's eyes. I definitely did not want to see what was going on.

"Is it supposed to bend that way?" Mom asked.

"I have to press down hard to get it in."

Mom sat down. The doctor removed the syringe, then repeated the maneuver on the other breast. When he was done, the nurse placed little bandages on each breast, then asked me to sit up slowly and take a deep breath. I did and felt nothing. Nothing at all! I felt exactly the same as I had before I got the fill. The procedure took all of five minutes. I got dressed and Mom and I walked out.

When we got to the waiting room, Mom said, "I have to sit down, Alana."

"What's the matter?"

"I feel woozy. I got all sweaty and queasy when they put those needles in."

"Oh, Mom!" I felt so bad. We sat quietly for a few minutes.

"I feel better now. We better get to your next appointment."

In the next waiting room, it seemed to take forever before we were called in. Again, a nurse asked me to disrobe and put on a gown, since my surgeon would want to look at my chest to see how it was healing. After I'd gotten changed, the nurse came back in. "You'll be happy to hear everything is good. The pathology results all came back negative for cancer."

"Sorry, can you repeat that?" I asked. I'd been expecting Doctor 7 to give us the results.

"The results showed no cancer cells in any of the tissue removed from your body."

"I'm cancer free?"

"Yes, congratulations!" She got ready to leave. "The doctor will be here in just a bit."

I couldn't talk for a minute. The day I had been diagnosed with breast cancer had been a turning point in my life, and now this day was one, too. I turned to my mother. "I'm cancer free!" I felt stunned, and yet I was ecstatic.

"I knew it! I knew everything would be okay. I'm so happy." But in a split second she went from beaming to frowning. "Are you upset that all your lymph nodes were removed?"

"Only to find out there wasn't any cancer in them? Not at all. I'd rather live my life without the nodes and be certain than have them spared and always wonder." I knew, regardless, that there was a need for checkups. "I know I'm more likely than the average person to get cancer again, but I'm happy I've done everything possible to get rid of it."

Doctor 7 came in then and clarified everything the nurse had said. "All of the lymph nodes that were taken out—nine in total—were negative for cancer. The cancerous lump margins were clear, and all of the remaining breast tissue that was removed was negative as well."

"Thank you," I said, grinning. What else could I say?

I was emotional, yet in many ways, I'd already experienced much more. I'd been on such a huge emotional roller-coaster ride over the past eight months, that these final results simply felt like a big relief.

Mom and I didn't say much when we left. I think we felt drained.

"All I want to do is make a few phone calls, grab some lunch, do some celebratory shopping the way we'd planned, and go home."

"Then that's exactly what we'll do."

"I want life to get back to normal again." For such a long time that was what I'd been thinking and hoping for, and now I was almost there. As I was getting ready for bed that night, I still felt fine—no soreness, no pressure on my chest. "I think I'm going to ask for 100 cubic centimeters at the next fill," I said to Greg. "I want to be bikini ready for the summer!"

Chapter 33

WHO ME, A SURVIVOR?

We arrived at the Relay for Life event early to get our tents and lawn chairs set up and register, even though everything didn't officially start until seven P.M.

"Look," I said to Adriana, "survivors get a special yellow T-shirt!" On the front it had the words *Celebrate, Remember, Fight Back*. Everyone else in the relay received a blue shirt with similar messages, so the yellow ones made us stand out. It was neat to be able to pick out my comrades in the crowd. I pulled on the shirt. With the initial fill I'd gotten during my surgery and the fill during my first appointment, it was starting to feel like I had breasts again. They were definitely different to the touch, but I had breasts and I was alive. I was happy.

Adriana told me that survivors would be kicking off the relay with a victory lap, which would be dedicated to all of the people who had been diagnosed with, conquered, or succumbed to cancer.

"I don't feel I belong to the survivors group."

"What are you talking about?" she said.

"I think I'm in denial somehow."

"Get out there!" She pushed me towards the starting line and the little group of about seven people wearing the yellow T-shirts. As I walked over, I realized that I recognized one of the survivors: a teenage boy named Brock. I used to babysit him when he was little. He'd been just ten months old when he was diagnosed with high-risk acute lymphoblastic leukemia. Because of her son's diagnosis, Brock's mother, Lori, had become a huge advocate for pediatric cancer patients and their families. She was a volunteer member of both the provincial and national public issue teams for the Canadian Cancer Society, worked to raise funds, and was also a national family advocate for the national caregiver advisory group in the Canadian Cancer Action Network. I was amazed by how she'd jumped into action when Brock had gotten ill. It was emotional to see him, because I never thought we'd be in the same situation, but it was inspiring, too, to see him alive and well sixteen years after all he'd gone through. If he could do it, so could I.

We started walking around the track, Brock and I beside each other, catching up on life and what his family had been up to since I had seen them last. I didn't notice it at first, or maybe I tried to block it out and distract myself so that I wouldn't get emotional, but the crowd of people who were watching and would take part after in the relay started cheering us, quietly at first, then louder and louder. I was startled. I started to cry and kept crying. I couldn't help but notice that a lot of other people were crying, too, including my group of girls. When we'd finished our victory lap, Lori presented the school with a plaque.

"Are you okay?" Adriana asked when I joined our team after the presentation.

"Yeah. It's weird, but I think that's the first time I identified myself as a cancer survivor. I've never thought about it that way before."

"It's cool."

"It is. They're all great people. But I hope one day everyone in the world will be in another group—the never-had-cancer group." I almost started crying again. "That we'll look back on this epidemic, and it will all be in the past—a part of history."

> "I think that's the first time I identified myself as a cancer survivor. I've never thought about it that way before."

Adriana hugged me.

"Cancer totally sucks," I said, and we started walking. The weather was rainy on and off, and windy, but everybody had such great energy that the weather couldn't keep our spirits down as we kept walking into the small hours of the night. "It's kind of strange, but I'm not that tired," I said to Adriana around three A.M. when we headed to our lawn chairs to have a bit of a break.

"Neither am I." She pulled out some cheese and crackers from the cooler she'd brought. "It must be the adrenaline of the whole thing."

"We'll be exhausted when we get home in a few hours for sure." Before long, we were up again—we knew that the longer we sat, the harder it would be to get back up. Before we knew it, we could see the sun starting to come up and could smell pancakes cooking. The walk ended at seven A.M., and by that time I was definitely exhausted.

"Thank you so much for organizing this, Adriana. I am so lucky to have such great friends!" I gave her and everyone else on our team a big hug. I was ready to go to bed—not for long, though. It was Sunday, and I wanted to hang out with the kids.

$\wp$

"Are you okay?" Mom asked on the following Tuesday morning. She'd walked into the kitchen as I was taking a pill.

"It's only a Tylenol. In case I feel pressure from the expansion." I was going for my second fill and planned to ask Doctor 9 to put in 100 cubic centimeters. I didn't have a clue how I'd feel after that.

"I've gotten Rudy dressed." My mom had bundled him up because even though it was May, it was an incredibly windy day and unusually cold.

"Great!" I said, but wondered if going alone would be easier. Mom would have to take care of Rudy anyway while Greg was working, since there weren't any day-care spots. "Are you sure you're okay coming, Mom? You have to do so much: get Rudy dressed, in and out of his car seat and stroller, and chase him around while I get filled up."

"I'm fine, Alana. Don't worry about me. You know I don't want you going to appointments alone."

I did like having someone with me, especially my mother, and I had to admit that I didn't know if I'd be able to drive home by myself, so along she came.

The drive was terrible. To say it was windy was an understatement. We'd just made it over the major skyway in our area when we heard on the radio it was being closed because of the gusts. I struggled to keep the car straight as the wind battered us from all sides. "Did you see that?" I said. "The windshield wiper got ripped off!" Next to go was a piece of rubber that sealed the front window. Something flew past, and I screamed, "What was that?"

"A ceiling tile, I think."

"They must be building houses nearby." A few pylons were strewn across the road near a section of construction. I navigated past them, then glanced anxiously at Rudy in the rearview mirror. We passed three transport trucks that had tipped over onto their sides on the opposite side of the highway.

"Are you sure we should keep going?" Mom asked as a roof shingle whipped past.

"We're almost there. If we turn back now, we'll have much farther to go." Somehow we made it to the appointment on time. "I guess our 'after-fill' shopping trip is out of the question," I said as we got out of the car.

Once inside, we had to wait quite a while. To distract Rudy, we chased him around in the hallway, then sat down to catch our breath.

"I've figured out how this setup works," I told Mom.

"What do you mean?" She looked confused.

"Since Doctor 9 sees so many patients, he has two operating rooms. See where the people have been going in and out?" Mom nodded. "While he's working on one, the nurses prep the next in the second room. Efficient."

We were called in. When Doctor 9 came in, he had a resident with him, whom he introduced, then he examined me. "How did the last fill go?"

"Great. In fact, so good with 60 cubic centimeters, I wanted to ask: Can I get more this time? I was thinking 120."

"That should be doable."

Doctor 9 took a syringe, prepped it, and began to push it into one breast, while the resident did the same with my other breast. They were tag-teaming me! I couldn't help but think, *Is this to save time? Is it so the resident can follow along?* I wasn't sure, but to be honest, I was fine with it because it took less time. It wasn't something I minded so much, but it certainly wasn't something I wanted to prolong. I sat up after the resident had put on the bandages. "My mind is saying, 'That should hurt like hell,' but my body isn't feeling a thing. Is that normal?"

"That's likely due to the lack of nerve connections from your previous surgeries," Doctor 9 said. "They do have the potential to repair themselves, but if they will remains to be seen."

Within fifteen minutes, I was done. I got dressed while Mom checked Rudy—luckily he'd fallen asleep in his stroller—and we were on our way down to the parking lot.

"How do you feel?" Mom asked.

"As the saline was injected, I felt a bit of pressure—mainly on the inside of my chest, as if the expanders were pressing in—but it didn't cause as much discomfort as I'd thought it would." I watched as she tucked Rudy into his car seat. "But it's weird walking into a room with your breasts one size, then walking out with them almost twice as big as they were before."

We set off. Thankfully the wind had died down.

"The beauty of reconstruction surgery done this way is that I can live with the results for two weeks, then decide if this size is just right or if I want to get bigger. I'm scheduled for two more fills, but I might not go for the last one—I don't want to get too big and live with backache for the rest of my life—but a perky C cup seems to be a nice way to finish off the journey."

"So this could be the last time you need to do this?"

"No. Even if I'm happy like this, I need one more fill—another 100 cubic centimeters in each breast in a few weeks."

"Why?"

"The skin needs to stretch a little more for the surgery. They need extra room to play with, so to speak. After that, we'd leave things for six more weeks so the skin can stretch for the final exchange surgery."

That night, Melanie came over to bring me some banana bread and rice pudding, which I loved. "How did it go today?"

"The drive was insane. We got home and found our barbecue had fallen over, and the kids' play set was blown clear across the pool! At least I didn't have to worry about my hair getting messed up by the wind!" I felt good enough now that I could joke about something like that. It was such a change from earlier days.

"It's really growing in, isn't it?"

"I even go out in public without my hat now."

"How does that feel?"

"Okay. I get looks from people I don't know, but I don't care. This is the longest my hair has been in a long time, so I want to show it off."

"Good for you!"

"I even wake up with bedhead sometimes, which is exciting. And I think I need to get my eyebrows sugared. I feel like an ape compared to a month ago!" And it was true. Maybe someone I didn't know wouldn't have noticed, and maybe I'd lived with my hair not growing for so long that it stood out to me, but it suddenly seemed as though my hair was coming back quicker than I thought it would. I went to visit Lepa every few weeks so she could shape it, and she wouldn't allow me to pay, just as she'd said at

HOLDING ON TO NORMAL

the haircutting party. My eyebrows and eyelashes were almost completely back to normal as well, and it had been only three months since I finished chemo. I had to start shaving my legs again, too. Never my favorite thing, but at this point I smiled every time I needed to do it. It was nice to have those leg hairs back.

Chapter 34

ON TRIAL

℘

*T**he plans for* our new house were coming along. I'd been researching different builders and had convinced Greg (and myself) that I could contract all of the trades out myself. It was a tough sell, but I knew it would be the most cost-effective route to go. He said yes on one condition: He didn't want anything to do with the process. So my days became consumed with architect appointments, phone calls trying to track down people to do the foundation, framing, drywall, insulation and roof, and everything in between. Not only that, of course, I had a few other things to think about as well.

"Are you going to sign up for the metformin trial?" Greg asked. With everything that had been going on, I hadn't committed to it, and he knew I had a year from my initial diagnosis to sign up for it and begin taking the drug.

"I think so." Helen, the clinical trial nurse, had said there would be few side effects, and I'd done more research and discovered that metformin had been around for years. "It's worth a try." But it was already May. I only had two months left to make the deadline. "I've filled out all of the paperwork, and I'm scheduled to have preliminary tests—X-rays and blood work. They need nine vials, apparently. They're going to drain me!"

"Why so many?"

"I don't know exactly, but I do know one of them is a pregnancy test. But that won't be a problem—after not having my period for four months while doing chemo, it's still quite irregular." I'd also experienced hot flashes and other menopausal symptoms, like night sweats and interrupted sleep, and that hadn't completely stopped yet, either. "With all of that, I'm pretty sure I'm not fertile, or pregnant."

"There's only one way to get pregnant," my mom said when I told her about the test.

I said, "I *know*, Mom," and rolled my eyes at her. What I didn't say was that during my brief experience with menopause, many things happened to my body that made intimacy the furthest thing from my mind. The random sweats made me feel gross, the hormone changes dried up certain places that never used to be dry, and I felt physically unattractive with my buzz cut and my wonky breasts. How on earth did women endure years of menopause? I knew one thing, though: the menopausal symptoms coupled with the trauma of my post-surgery body made it virtually impossible for a pregnancy to even come close to happening. I just didn't want to get into all of that with my mom.

I needed to go to JCC to have my blood taken for the trial, as well as get the necessary X-rays. I dropped the kids off at day care and picked up my mom, and we headed off to the hospital. I probably could have taken my kids with me to this appointment, but honestly how much fun would it be for them to sit in the car for an hour on the way there, wait in the waiting room while I had X-rays and blood work for who knows how long, and then sit in the car again for an hour on the way back. The day care was a godsend. I loved it and so did the kids.

When we arrived at JCC, the first stop was the lab. As promised, they drew nine vials of blood. I had been doing this so often that the needles didn't bother me one bit anymore—I was so used to being poked and prodded.

At the X-ray clinic, I was checked in and given a gown by the technician. "Remove your bra and shirt, please, then put this on. I'll be back in a minute," she said. When I was finished changing, she returned and led me into a room. "Stand here," she said, and positioned me properly before she moved behind a window nearby. "Take a deep breath and hold it," she said. I could hear the machine click once, then stop. The technician came out from behind the glass. "Do you have anything inside you?"

For a second, I wondered what she meant. "Oh, yes, expanders, for breast reconstruction."

"I wondered what those were."

I almost started laughing, she looked so confused. "Can I see what they look like?"

"Sure." She waved me behind the window and pointed at a computer monitor. "That's you."

"They look so funny!" On the screen was what appeared to be a normal-looking chest X-ray, except for two circles side by side that looked like bullet holes. "No wonder you looked so perplexed when you asked!"

After the X-ray was done, Mom and I headed up to the clinical trials office.

"I wonder if I'm going to get metformin or a placebo."

"I hope it's the metformin."

When Helen arrived, she invited us to sit down, then said, "We have a problem."

"What?" I swallowed hard. "It hasn't even been six months since I finished chemo . . ." The only thing I could think would be a problem was that they found some kind of sign indicating a recurrence of cancer in my blood work.

"No, no, there's nothing wrong," Helen said. "But your HCG levels, the hormone that indicates pregnancy, are elevated."

"What?"

She studied her papers. "Your HCG level is at two, and we need it to be at one in order to continue with the study. We need to be certain you're not pregnant."

"I'm positive I'm not."

"I'm afraid we can't go by that. The only way we can be sure is for you to take another pregnancy test in a few days. If you are pregnant, that number would double every twenty-four to seventy-two hours. If you're not, then it will remain the same or go back down to one."

"Has this happened before?" Mom asked.

"I'm afraid not."

Of course, I thought. It had to happen to me.

I laughed a little, as I glanced at my mother, but I didn't think it was funny at all. I wanted to be part of the trial. I wanted that drug. I tried to think of something else.

$\wp$

"I can't believe it's time for a checkup already." I still had to meet with Doctor 7, my oncologist, before we could go home.

"The time has gone so quickly," my mother said.

"It has! But look, here's a marker." I ran a hand through my hair. It wasn't particularly even all over, despite Lepa's efforts, but if I pulled on it, I could stretch it to about an inch. It was coming in a bit coarser than before, with a slight wave to it, and in certain lights it looked almost salt and pepper as opposed to my old blond color.

"It's looking so cute."

"It is, isn't it?"

By the time we got to Doctor 7's office, the talk had distracted me somewhat, but I was wondering how the hell I could be pregnant.

Doctor 7 examined me. "You have a little redness underneath your left breast. If it gets very red, let me know. That could be a sign of cellulitis, a common skin infection caused by bacteria. But otherwise everything seems fine. Before you go, though, I want to run through the major symptoms of a recurrence you need to be aware of."

"Just a minute," I said and got out my notebook.

"Ready? Sudden persistent headache, unusual lumps, a strange cough that doesn't go away, trouble breathing, pain in your bones that's persistent and unexplainable."

"I know I've been told, but I have to ask again, what are the odds of a recurrence?"

"You have about a 40 percent chance of recurrence."

My face fell.

"Your chances of recurrence were 60 percent before chemotherapy," she said gently, "and chemotherapy reduces the risk by about a third."

I left the office feeling rather subdued. "I'm more determined than ever to get into the metformin trial," I said to my mother. "I can't stop thinking about that number—forty. It's so high."

"You're doing everything you possibly can to keep cancer at bay, Alana. If you look at it differently, you have a 60 percent chance of it not coming back." I wanted to do everything possible to change those percentages, but it frustrated me that some things I couldn't change. I could participate in the trial, I could eat healthy, I could be on alert for the signs of recurrence, but I just couldn't change those numbers. I felt helpless.

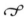

First, though, I would have to find out if I was pregnant. Four days later I went to the lab closest to my home to have a pregnancy test done. It took twenty-four hours for the results to come back. Helen called when they did. My HCG level was less than five, but that's as precise as they got. The level could have been one, two, three or four for that matter, but their machine wasn't high tech enough to get numbers smaller than five, so the results weren't accurate enough.

"It would be best if you get a blood test at JCC," Helen said. She suggested I wait another two weeks and get it on the same day that I had my fill appointment. By then we would know for sure by the numbers whether or not I was indeed pregnant.

The two weeks went by, and Greg and Mom joked about the situation quite a bit, but we were the only people in on the joke. We decided that it probably wouldn't be wise to tell everyone about this little glitch in the plan. I honestly didn't believe I was, but . . . that was something I didn't want to think about. I loved being a mom. I loved my kids to pieces. I lived for them, and I had never imagined the happiness that they would bring me. Every once in a while, Charley would ask if she could have a sister. (It was kind of funny that she never asked if she could have another brother, but I guess that's probably how older sisters feel about younger brothers.)

My answer was always the same: "Mommy has so much love for both you and Rudy that I don't want to share it. I don't want to share my love with anyone else. It's all for the both of you." The real fact of the matter was that they both made me happy, and I didn't feel the need to add more to the mix. We were good.

Being diagnosed with cancer and going through all the chemotherapy I went through took a toll on my body, not to mention my reproductive organs. I'd gone through early menopause, after all. What effect had all of that had on my eggs? I was approaching thirty-five, too. I knew that there were more health risks involved for both the baby and me. Not to mention, I'd had cancer while I was breastfeeding. Did the pregnancy cause or encourage the cancer to grow? The doctors didn't say it had, but they also never said that it hadn't. Oh, and let's not forget, I didn't have any breasts left. I wouldn't be able to breastfeed.

My body simply wasn't in tiptop shape. I'd been lucky to have survived this time around, but I didn't want to do anything that would put my future health or a baby's health at risk. And if I was pregnant, I definitely wouldn't be able to be on the metformin trial. There would be no more babies in my future, I had decided, and I was fine with that. I had two beautiful healthy kids, and I was on my way to being healthy as well. I felt no need to mess with that.

I talked to Greg. "Greg, you know if the test was positive, we'd have a big decision to make."

"I know. Ultimately, that's something we would have to think about. But for right now the test isn't positive," he said, trying to reassure me.

"I know, but it's not negative."

"Try not to think about it until you go for your next test. I'm sure it's just a glitch."

I nodded. It *was* just a glitch. I remembered what my mom said. There was only one way to get pregnant.

Finally two weeks had passed. The swelling from the surgery had gone down, and I at last had a truer sense of the size of my breasts. They were bigger than they'd ever been, but I was comfortable with them, and wanted to keep them this size. So I decided to go for that final fill of an extra 100 cubic centimeters, and headed out for my appointments, which were at two different hospitals: one for the fill, and the other at JCC for the blood work results.

When we arrived at the first hospital, though, it was to the sound of fire alarms. I shook my head and thought, *My whole cancer experience has been nothing but drama, and now there are fire alarms on top of everything!*

"What's happening?" I asked one of the people gathered outside.

"We're not sure, but the entire hospital is on lockdown."

"We're going to be late," I said to my mother, worried I'd miss my appointment.

"So is everyone," Mom pointed out.

"True."

Mom was right. When we got to the office we were ushered right in to an exam room, the receptionist saying, "We've already seen everyone else who was up here while the lockdown was taking place."

Doctor 9 was pleased with my progress. "Your breasts are healing well."

"I'm really happy with them. But I think the right breast is slightly larger than the left."

Doctor 9 stood back and looked at me. "I think you're right. Not to worry, we'll add a bit more to your left breast today." Once again, he and a resident injected both breasts at the same time, and Mom and I were on our way in fifteen minutes.

I tugged at my bra as we got in the car, on our way to the next appointment. "It's weird. Even though I didn't feel any discomfort before, today I do."

"Maybe you're getting some feeling back?"

"You're right. Could be the nerves are reconnecting the way they said they might. Or maybe there's just more pressure now because my breasts are bigger. The implant doesn't have anywhere to go until the skin has a chance to stretch. Anyway, if that's what it is, I know it'll stop in a few days."

I strapped myself in and started driving off almost before Mom had a chance to do the same. I was driving. I knew I'd be okay doing it and I wanted to get to JCC as fast as possible for my blood work.

"Why the rush?" Mom asked.

"Because I'll likely have to wait a while for the results, and I have to meet Helen to get the metformin after." We managed to make it to the lab just after 10:45 A.M. Luckily there weren't too many people there, so I got my blood drawn just before eleven. Then we went in search of Helen.

When we found her at the clinical studies office, I told her, "The blood is on its way to the lab."

"Great. I'll ask for a quick turnaround, too." She called. "They say it'll be at least an hour before we hear anything, so you might want to grab lunch."

"Sounds like a good plan." Mom and I had a quick bite in the cafeteria, then were headed to pick up the chest X-rays I'd ordered (I thought it would be fun to have a copy of the films with the expanders) when my phone rang. I looked to see who it was.

"It's Helen," I said to Mom. It had been only about forty-five minutes since I'd had my blood drawn.

"The results came back showing an error," she said. "They have to be done again."

"Seriously?" I made a face at Mom. This was getting nutty.

"You don't have to have more blood taken, though. The lab will test the blood they have again."

I ended the call. We went back to the cafeteria, drank endless cups of coffee, and of course, people-watched. The wait was excruciating. After two hours and counting, my phone rang again. Mom started asking what was said before I even hung up.

"I'm not pregnant!"

"That's wonderful."

"That's a different reaction from the last two times I was pregnant," I joked.

She laughed. "I'm so happy you can go on the drug now."

"Me too. I mean, as much as I love my kids, this is the best news I could have gotten."

I texted Greg to tell him the news as we practically ran out of the cafeteria to meet Helen at the pharmacy.

"I've placed the order for you," she said. "It should be ready in a minute. It's a six-month supply of metformin or placebo." She had barely finished talking and the pharmacist was already calling my name.

We thanked Helen, picked up the package and left. I wanted to get home so I could take the metformin, if that's what it was. And whatever it was, I would be taking it for the next five years.

Chapter 35

FINAL SURGERY

$\mathcal{P}$

I was obsessed with trying to find out if I was taking the "actual" pill or just the placebo. The pharmacist had given me a glucose meter—one of those little gadgets that pricks your finger to draw a drop of blood—that diabetics use to test their blood sugar levels, and I was convinced that I could use it to figure out which I was on. I'd been on the pills for about a week, and I was dying to know what exactly they were.

"What are you doing?" Mom asked me when she saw me with the meter.

"I'm going to test my blood sugar. Then I'll eat lunch, test it again, take a pill and test it one more time. I want to see if the pill is making my sugar levels drop." She watched me prick my finger and check the numbers.

"What does it say?"

"Eighty-four."

"What does that mean?"

"I don't know!" We both burst out laughing. I had no idea at all what I was doing, and realized figuring it out might not be as easy as I thought. But I went ahead and tested my blood sugar again immediately after I'd eaten something, and the meter read 81. I took a pill, waited about fifteen minutes and tested my blood again, and the number was 79.

"What is it at now?" Mom asked, about half an hour after lunch. I pricked my finger and it was back to 80. "What does that mean?"

"I have no clue." I had no idea what any of the numbers meant. The whole thing was beyond my area of expertise.

"Whatever it is you're taking, you can't change that." I think she sensed my frustration. "Try to believe that it *is* metformin, and try not to stress about it. Let's think about something else. How are the house plans coming?"

"Overwhelming as well." I'm not sure she realized how that was stressful, too. But I was the one who'd chosen to be so busy. And the house was keeping me occupied, which was the point, wasn't it? "I was getting quotes for foundations, and I honestly think they're jacking the price up because they think I'm a rookie and don't know what I'm doing."

Mom gave me a look. "You know I'm the first to support you in whatever you do. You know that. But maybe this is a little over your head. There's a lot you could mess up, and it's a lot of work. What happens when you go back to work in September? How are you going to juggle work and kids and building a house all by yourself? Why are you putting so much on your plate?" Even though it sounded blunt, I knew she was being cautious about the words she chose.

"I know. I just wanted to save some money."

"You just went through a major illness. Your health is important. Your stress levels are important. Think about leaving this in the hands of someone who knows what they are doing. Not that you couldn't," she said hurriedly. "I believe you can do anything you set your mind to. I just don't think you need the added stress right now."

"I feel sort of empowered doing it, like nothing can stop me. Like I can do anything."

"You can! Just pick something that's not going to cause you so much stress. Write a book! And build a smaller house if you want to save money."

She had made a lot of good points and usually didn't voice her opinions to this extent. Maybe I needed to shift my focus, downsize our plan a bit. My well-being was important, and now that I had a clean bill of health, I needed to keep it that way.

Mom was right. I cut some square footage off the plan, eliminating areas we didn't need. I agreed to hire a builder and started looking around town to check out the work the ones I had in mind had done. I even set up meetings to price out the design. The meetings would take place after my surgery, of course, but in the meantime, that planning kept me busy. And I knew that because I was so busy, it would be time for the operation before I knew it.

℘

The day of the exchange surgery arrived. It had been a few weeks since I had started taking the metformin. I was feeling good and was ready for this next step.

"Are you nervous?" Greg asked.

"Not at all. I'm excited."

"Excited? It's surgery."

"I know, but this one is different. After the lumpectomy, I had to wait to find out what grade, stage and type of tumor was growing inside of me. After the mastectomy, I had to wait to find out if the margins were clear and if everything was gone." I shrugged. "This time there's none of that. It's just surgery. No results. No life-or-death outcomes. When I leave the hospital, I'll be officially finished with everything." I didn't say it out loud, but I was mentally and emotionally exhausted. I was physically ravaged.

I looked at Greg. "I'm so ready to be done."

✐

I felt like a pro when I arrived for surgery this time.

"I know the whole routine," I said to Greg. "How weird is that? It shouldn't be that way, should it?"

"No, not at all." He left to get a coffee while the nurses did their thing. He knew this prepping process would take a bit of time, and figured he'd get out of everyone's way. After I'd been prepped, Doctor 9, the plastic surgeon, came by and asked how I was doing.

"I wish this was all over, but otherwise good."

"That's understandable, but before you know it, we'll be finished. Right now I'm going to mark where things need to be on you, starting by defining the center line of your chest." He pulled out a black marker and began drawing on me, which tickled somewhat—I didn't have all of the sensation back, but I could feel what he was doing a little. "Now I'm marking where the bottom of your new breasts will be, and the outer edges." He then wrote on my left arm. "This is a note to remind everyone involved not to use this arm for blood-pressure monitoring."

He was finishing up when another doctor came in. He explained he was a resident. "I'm here to double-check your charts and find out what pain relief you prefer."

"Percocet," I said before he even offered a choice.

"Percocet, it is." Both Doctor 9 and the resident left, and an anesthesiologist and his resident arrived.

"My job is to make sure you don't feel a thing," the anesthesiologist explained. "I'm going to administer just enough anesthesia that you'll be asleep during the entire surgery, which will last about one and a half hours."

"Best sleep ever, right?"

"That's one way to think of it. Can you open your mouth wide for me, please?"

"What? Why?"

"I just need to check that there's room should I need to insert a breathing tube."

Visualizing myself on the operating table with a tube down my throat scared me. I tried to shake the thought. It occurred to me that it would be best for me to stop asking questions I didn't want the answers to.

Greg returned with his coffee. I said to him, "It's reassuring but kind of nerve-racking realizing how many doctors are involved in a surgery like this. Honestly, it's starting to feel like a parade. And for some reason I thought that the last time the anesthesia I was given was a type of gas I breathed in. But apparently that was just oxygen—what knocked me out was what was in the IV."

"They didn't tell you that last time?"

"I don't think so. But the anesthesiologist also said a tube might need to be stuck down my throat to help me breathe. I remember having a sore throat last time and wondering why. So maybe they did need to stick it down my throat?" I didn't want to even imagine that. Before I could freak out further, a nurse came to walk me to the operating room. Greg kissed me good-bye.

"I feel as though we've been playing out this same scene way too many times."

"You'll be done after this," he said and squeezed my hand.

I tried to focus on what Greg said when I lay down on the operating table. I was shivering again from both the cold and nerves. I couldn't help myself—I may have gone through this before, but that didn't mean I wasn't scared.

The anesthesiologist placed the oxygen mask over my mouth, and he must have started the IV, because I began to feel less anxious. The next thing I knew, I woke up in the recovery room. I dozed in and out of sleep, and in between, the nurses checked my vitals, offered me small sips of water, and came by to see if I needed anything. After about an hour in recovery, I was wheeled back to the ward, where Greg was waiting.

"Hey, how are you feeling? Better or worse than last time?" he asked.

"After my mastectomy it felt as though there were elephants sitting on my chest, but this time it feels different. There's definitely some pain, but it's less intense and the pressure isn't there."

"That's great. Maybe this will be a better experience all around."

I hoped he was right.

When I felt better, I was allowed to get dressed. A nurse removed my IV and rechecked my vitals. She said I was free to go as long as I was up to it. I knew I was, and just like that, an hour and a half after surgery ended, we were on our way home.

When we got there, the kids were there to greet me, and so was my mom, blocking them from trying to jump all over me. She looked tired. She must have been exhausted with the stress of worrying about me, and with coping with Charley's and Rudy's bursts of energy. Despite that, she was anxious to help me.

"Come in and sit down. Let me help you with your shoes. What can I do?"

"It's okay, Mom. Honestly, it's better this time."

"Please don't overdo it. It was surgery. You have to take care of yourself." She glanced at me, and I knew she meant business.

I ended up feeling as exhausted as she probably was. I crashed on the couch, and by the time Greg sent the kids to kiss me good night so he could put them to bed, I decided I needed to follow suit. I'd made it till almost eight o'clock and that was late enough.

"How are you, Alana?" Mom asked when she saw me go by. "You don't look so good."

"Okay, except for this nagging feeling of nausea I just can't seem to shake." I almost made it to bed, but had to run into the master bathroom, where I threw up in the sink.

My mom came running. "Don't worry about it. Just go up to bed. I'll clean up."

"I'm so sorry. I just couldn't make it to the toilet."

After she was done, she came and wiped my face with a washcloth.

"The nurses told me not to eat large amounts of food, and I didn't, but whatever I ate didn't mix well with the anesthetic lingering in my body."

"That happens. Lots of people get sick from the anesthetic."

"I'm going to take a Percocet. I hope that will help me get through the night." I closed my eyes.

That Percocet was a godsend. I took another one in the night but slept for nine hours. I'd probably been overly optimistic after the operation. I'd thought it would be a piece of cake compared to everything else.

The worst thing about surgery was the constant lethargy for a few days afterwards. "I feel as though I'm sleeping constantly," I said to Melanie when I called her a couple of days later at school. "The first day I took three naps, and today I've taken two so far, even though it's only the afternoon."

"I guess it's your body's way of telling you to rest."

"That makes sense. I guess it's just the effects of the anesthesia wearing off, and just surgery in general. I'm so glad Mom is here to help out with the kids again. I'm sore—not as bad as the last time—but I can't lift anything."

"I am making banana bread tonight, so I'll try to swing by with some tomorrow after school. In the meantime, get your butt to bed, will ya?"

I laughed. She always cheered me up. "Thanks, Mel. And yes, I will."

As I hung up, Mom came into the living room with the kids to announce that they were going to the park.

"Mommy, it's time for your nap," Charley said, and she pulled a blanket over me and gave me a kiss. I must have fallen asleep almost instantly, because when I woke up, they were back home, with my mom trying to get dinner ready.

I was taking Percocet—it helped with the pain—but the days began to blur together and speed by because of the frequent naps. Often before I knew it, it was almost bedtime and I was sitting on the couch with the kids reading a bedtime story.

One night, as I sat there with the two of them snuggled up next to me, I looked down. I thought Charley had spilled water on me.

"Oh, crap," I said.

"What is it?" Greg asked.

"I think a drain must be leaking." I got up. "I'm going to check." I didn't want to alarm the kids, so Greg continued with the story where I'd left off.

I went to the master bathroom and took off my shirt. There was a large reddish circle underneath my armpit. I called the home-care nurse.

"Hi, it's Alana. Something's wrong," I said and explained the situation.

"I'll come right over."

Greg came in. "What's going on?"

"The nurse is going to do an emergency house call."

I soaked through two more shirts by the time the nurse was able to come. She had a look. "I'll patch you up to get you through the night."

"Great." I was relieved that she was going to be able to do something. "The drains have been pinching me every time I move."

"Hmm. They shouldn't be doing that."

"It's not too bad, it just feels a little bit like tape being removed from a hairy arm. I figured that the drain was wedging itself in between my breast and rib cage."

She looked more closely at them. "This one doesn't have much gauze around it, and it was partially clogged with a blood clot. I'm going to change the dressing, and I've milked the drain to get rid of the clot." She took care of everything and packed up her supplies. "Call me back if you have any other problems and when the drains are producing less than 30 cubic centimeters of fluid in less than twenty-four hours, so I can come back to remove them."

Fortunately, the drains didn't leak again. For the next few days, it was business as usual, if usual business consisted of milking drains and taking sponge baths. I played with the kids in and around the house to make the time go faster, but didn't go too far because of the drains. Luckily the weather was beautiful outside, so we could play in the backyard. I also kept myself occupied with plans for the new house while getting ready to list ours. I showed Greg a draft plan that I'd received from an architect.

"It's three thousand square feet. Don't you think it's too big?"

"You can't take it with you," he said, referring to the money we'd be spending on it. "And there's not much we can take out. Let's just do it."

"I'm pricing out some things. Maybe we should wait a bit. Who knows what's going to happen with me." That was my fear talking, fear that I wasn't going to make it.

"You'll be fine, Alana. Don't worry. Let's list our house and start digging the second it sells."

I wasn't totally convinced, but at least I was busy for a while.

∽

I was so excited four days after my surgery when the home-care nurse pulled in our driveway.

"These drains will never be a part of my life again," I said to Greg. "But I think getting them out is going to hurt this time, because of that pinching feeling I had."

"If it does, I'm sure it will last less than a couple seconds, kind of like a bandage coming off. Once it's done I'm sure you won't feel a thing."

"I hope so," I said as I went to the door to let her in.

The nurse unpacked her supplies and ran through the same routine as the last time while I got myself comfortable on the bed. She counted down and I took a deep breath, bracing myself, but she was so quick, she had to tell me when each one was out.

When it was over, I said, "Thank you so much. You were great," and sat up, quickly pulling on my shirt. I wasn't trying to rush her out, but Greg and I walked her to the front door to show her out. As she left, I said to Greg, "I feel as though each time I close a door on someone like that, I'm moving on with my life."

And I was. We were. I went downstairs to e-mail an update.

Hey, everyone!

I'm done! The exchange surgery is over, the expanders are out, and my breasts look amazing. I am so happy with the way it all went. We all are. In fact, I'm going to have a drink to celebrate.

I hit send, then stared at the screen. I'd sat in front of this computer for so many hours, wondering what was going to happen to me, looking up statistics, scribbling down numbers, doing everything I could to try to get control. I thought, *Am I really here? Is it over?* I stood up and shook myself.

It was.

The house actually went up for sale a few weeks later in the summer. In fact, we listed it and it sold within a couple of weeks to the first person who looked at it. We then gave the builder the green light to go ahead and start building our new house, since the closing date for our old house was in February 2012, and we needed to get moving—literally.

Chapter 36

FINISHING TOUCHES

$\mathcal{P}$

I was thinking about nipples all the time: having them, not having them.

"Charley is four years old and curious," I said to my mother. "Before I had breast cancer, she saw my breasts all the time. I didn't make a point of covering up when she walked into the bathroom after I got out of the shower, and three-year-olds definitely don't knock before entering. I was also breastfeeding Rudy when she was with me a lot! But now my breasts have changed, and I don't want her to be frightened by that. She's too young to understand the complexity of it all."

"Has she said anything to you yet?"

"No, but she hasn't seen them lately. I've been trying to cover up my chest so she doesn't." I wasn't sure yet what the right approach to take was.

"Why don't you just keep yourself covered if you don't feel comfortable with her seeing you like this?"

"I don't want to always feel the need to cover up if she walks into the bathroom or whatever. Someday she's going to know everything that happened to me. I need to decide what I'm going to do. Originally, I thought I wanted to have a nipple-creating surgery, which I could do if I wanted. But now I'm not so sure." To create a nipple, skin from each breast would have to be cut, pulled together, and then tied. An areola would then be tattooed on to create a natural look. "I was talking with some girlfriends and they mentioned the possibility of a 3-D nipple. I think that might be the better route for me."

"Have you talked to Greg about it?" she asked.

"I did talk, and he was supportive of whatever decision I made, but said it needed to be my decision. He said he didn't care if I had nipples or not, which is nice, but it's hard having to make so many decisions on my own."

"What are the pros and cons of each option?"

"I guess it boils down to having a nipple that protrudes. With surgery, my nipples will always stick out. With tattoos, they never will but might look like they are, because the tattoos are 3-D."

"That seems simple to me then. With the tattoos you can have the best of both worlds."

I agreed. I realized I'd just needed some validation, so I felt as though I was making the right decision.

I began looking into the 3-D tattoos, and discovered there was a medical tattoo artist a few hours away from me who specialized in micropigmentation and nipple tattoos. I called her up.

"It's a process of inserting color pigments underneath the skin in layers," the artist explained, "which is different from regular tattooing. Because it's layered, it creates a 3-D effect. The needles I use go into the skin at different depths to help me get exactly the right look."

"It was fascinating," I told Greg after the call. "I was so impressed by what she had to say, I've decided to meet with her."

"If that's what you want. You have to be happy."

My appointment was at the end of August. The artist's name was Kyla, and her office was located in a medical building in Peterborough. I was happy to discover that she worked in conjunction with a plastic surgeon—I figured her work must be good if that was the case—and the reception area and waiting room were for both practices. When I arrived, the receptionist had me fill out a questionnaire about my medical history. Then I got to talk with Kyla, who soon put me at ease. I couldn't wait to ask her how she got into this line of work.

"I studied art at Oxford and became a professor. But when I was twenty-seven, I was diagnosed with ovarian cancer." She explained that because of chemotherapy, she was left with no eyebrows and lost much of the pigmentation in her lips. While she was in the hospital, a nurse offered to tattoo her eyebrows, but because the nurse wasn't very artistic she was left with asymmetrical purple eyebrows. A permanent makeup artist then offered to fix her brows and add pigment to her lips. But the pigments caused severe allergic reactions and had to be cut out.

I was stunned by her story and not surprised when she said, "I became dedicated to researching the latest advancements in medical tattoos and helping patients like you." She showed me pictures of her work. It was amazing—it all looked so real. I went home and called my mother. "I'm ecstatic about the idea of this. It's so much less invasive than surgery, and it looks so realistic. I've booked my appointments already."

"How many are there, and when is the first one?"

"The first is in October—I need to make sure that the swelling from surgery has completely gone down before I go. Then I'll have another one four weeks later."

October was a couple of months away. I couldn't wait, but so much would be happening by then: I would be well into teaching the new year of school, Charley would be starting her first year of school, and construction on our new house would be well under way. By the end of August the foundation was dug, the framing had begun, and the doors and windows were on their way.

Charley was definitely ready to start school, and I was ready to go back

as well. Getting into a routine would be good for everyone. It would be
hectic, though. Lunches would need to be packed the night before. I would
have to get the kids ready to leave the house by 7:45 each morning, drive
about fifteen minutes to Rudy's day care, and then another fifteen minutes
from the day care to school. That would leave me some time in the morning to get prepped for class but not much, since I'd have Charley with me
for a while, too, before she headed over to her classroom. After school we'd
have to pick Rudy up, drive home, unpack everything, get dinner ready,
have baths. Then after the kids went to bed, we'd start the whole thing over
again.

As it turned out, I was right about the routine. It was good. School was
going well, but any free time I had after the kids went to bed was spent
focusing on the new house. I was exhausted, but the time flew by.

$\wp$

Mom came with me to the first tattoo appointment. I had no idea what to
expect. I'd never had a tattoo. A friend who had one had told me, "It feels
kind of like tiny little pinches. Not so much throbbing pain but irritating."
Even so, I was nervous.

When we arrived at Kyla's office, everyone was just starting to come
back from their lunch breaks, and things were quite quiet. When she was
ready for us, I swiftly realized that she was a perfectionist.

"I need you to sit up straight so I can draw with a marker where I am
going to start the tattoos."

"How do you even figure that out?"

"Ideally we want them to sit slightly lower than center so they look natural, and the nipples themselves should be mirror images of each other." As
she explained that, she showed me how she'd used an inkblotting trick to
replicate the image of the first nipple that she'd drawn onto the other side.
Although we kept chatting, she was completely focused on her work. She
was meticulous about everything. After we were both completely satisfied

with the potential size and location of the new nipples, it was time to start tattooing.

"It feels so weird," I said to Kyla as she began. It didn't hurt, but it also wasn't a pleasant feeling. I still didn't have much feeling in my chest, but my friend was right: it did feel like tiny little pinches. Every so often Kyla would stand back, take a look and add more ink in certain spots, switch colors on the machine, change needles, wipe away blood and then continue. After almost two hours, she got up and called me over to the other side of the room, where there was a full-length mirror.

"Well, what do you think?" she asked.

I stood in front of the mirror, new nipples staring me straight in the face. Although the freshly inked tattoos looked a little red, they were uncanny. "Wow. That is incredible. They look so real!"

"I don't want you to get them wet. Here are enough supplies to last you a week," she said, handing me a care package filled with gauze and ointment, as well as a detailed instruction sheet on how to care for my new nipples. It sounded kind of funny: *my new nipples.*

It was a long drive home. I was excited to get back and show everyone, which also was kind of funny. Never before I had cancer had I wanted to show anyone my breasts, and never before did anyone want to see them. I'd never even worn clothing that was too revealing, but if any part of my breasts were ever exposed at all, my nipples certainly weren't. That was taboo, culturally, wasn't it? You'd see cleavage in magazines, but never nipples. But this was different—these weren't actually my nipples. They were fake—in essence, pictures of nipples—so I had no problem showing them to anyone. I still felt almost separated from them, so it was no big deal in a way. All of my friends were curious, and I was happy to oblige. And the responses all made me very happy.

"Wow, they look so real!" Melanie said as I pulled her into the bathroom at work to show her.

"That's just crazy," Erin said when I showed her at my parents' house one Sunday evening.

"Are you kidding me?" another friend, Kristy, said when I showed her in the washroom stall of a restaurant where we were having dinner one night.

It became quite comical. But the best part was that the tattoos weren't even finished yet.

Four weeks later, I went for the second appointment, and again my mom tagged along. I came out with my nipples looking even more real than they had the last time, which, if you'd asked me prior to the appointment, would have seemed virtually impossible. Kyla's attention to detail astounded me.

I walked out of her office feeling finished somehow: I had my new breasts, I had new nipples. I knew I had to go for checkups—somehow in the back of my mind, I knew that this would never be over—but for now I was done. And not only did my new nipples look real, they made me feel like a real person again. *Whole*—that was difficult for people to understand. For a woman, losing her breasts and having her hair fall out changes everything, and damages—if it doesn't destroy—her self-esteem. I was a fairly confident woman before I was diagnosed with cancer, and I wish I could have said that I was stronger than that, and that I wouldn't be affected by losing my hair and my breasts, but the reality is, I wasn't invincible.

> I knew that this would never be over—but for now I was done. And not only did my new nipples look real, they made me feel like a real person again. *Whole.*

❧

My brother and I hadn't chatted much throughout my whole ordeal. We joked back and forth quite a bit when we did, and it occurred to me that maybe that was his way of handling the situation. Shortly after my second tattoo session, he called to check in on me.

"How are things?"

"Good. Busy. It's tough getting back into the swing of things with work."

"Don't you think you've been milking this thing for too long?" he said.

I knew he wasn't serious, but I couldn't wait to put him in his place—that's what sisters do, right?

"Would you like to trade places?"

Silence. He had no response.

Chapter 37

A GIFT FROM THE HEART

ॐ

*U*ncle *Jimmy, my* mom's eldest brother, hadn't seen me at all since my haircutting party, but he knew I'd had a rough time during chemo. He was just one of about fifteen people who came over to my parents' house for Thanksgiving dinner. It was the usual big family gathering, and as always, Mom had made way too much food—at least enough to feed thirty. Erin and her kids, Natalie and Jack, were there, and Charley and Rudy had a blast playing with them, as always.

When we managed to corral the kids to sit down to eat, I looked around the dinner table and couldn't help but think about everything that had happened over the past months and what I had gone through to be there that night. Many of the people sitting at the table had been a part of my journey. Rudy was the person closest to me when I found the lump on what turned out to be such a fateful night. My mom and Greg were there with me at the exact time that I heard the devastating announcement that I had cancer. My dad, who had turned up crying on my doorstep, was now sitting with me at dinner, looking forward to a great evening in my company, something he probably hadn't thought he was going to be able to do for very much longer. My uncle Jimmy had shaved his head in solidarity with me at the haircutting party.

I could see Charley's eyes widen when the turkey was brought out. She had the gift of being excited about everything. She'd thought my hair looked great when it was cut off, and was thrilled to put barrette after barrette in it after it started growing back. She was my constant caregiver, always checking in to see how Mommy was doing, never disillusioned by anything, whether it be my appearance or my bald head. She was ready and willing to do anything. That was the way she was. And Erin and her husband, Doug, had both taken me to chemo treatments, and Jack and Natalie had made me signs and cupcakes for my last chemo treatment.

Everyone around that table had been with me every step of the way, and they were there with me still. With their help, I had survived. I'd always felt thankful for many things, but this year, giving thanks had special meaning.

After dinner, when we were all getting ready to leave, Uncle Jimmy pulled me aside. We hadn't had much of a chance to talk during the meal, and he told me how good I looked.

"You sound surprised, Uncle Jimmy."

"I suppose I am. I expected you to be weak and frail." He bowed his head and said, "I brought you something."

"What's wrong, Uncle Jimmy?"

"It's just . . . What I thought might have been appropriate a while back may not be that appropriate anymore, but I want to give it to you because I made it myself." Whatever it was, was in his car, so he went out to go get it while I waited near the front door. When he came back inside, he handed me a handmade wooden cane stained a gorgeous shade of pale pink.

"It's beautiful." I was so touched by the obvious thought and care that had gone into the gift.

"I hand-carved and hand-stained it."

I could tell how awkward he felt, realizing only now that I didn't need a cane.

"It's the best gift ever, Uncle Jimmy!" I hugged him. I meant it. "When I turn ninety and need a cane to walk with, this is the cane I'll use. Do you mind if I show everyone?" He nodded and grinned. I knew he was pleased.

Everyone loved the cane. As they passed it around, I thought about how things were changing. I could eat a normal meal again without worrying about throwing up. The copious drugs that had been consumed or pumped into my body were out of my system. My hair was growing back, and my eyelashes and eyebrows, too. As time went by, life was becoming more and more normal. But being a breast cancer survivor would always be my new normal. Some things would never go back to the way they were. I would always have scars—inside and out. I would never have my old breasts back. Yet I was happy. Whenever I looked at my new breasts, I felt that I was one of the lucky ones, lucky enough to have gotten through this journey and made it to the other side.

Uncle Jimmy handed the cane back to me. I took it and felt how strong it was. I knew that it would last through the years and hold me up when I got old. As I held it, I thought, *Happily ever after.* And I knew that although my journey in life had already taken me down some dark paths, there were also lovely surprises. And my life was carrying on.

EPILOGUE

There were days on this journey that were horrible—unthinkably so. The worst days were those surrounding my diagnosis, the first days of my hair loss, and those extremely nauseating times during my first four rounds of chemo. To say that those days scarred me would be an understatement. But there weren't many moments when I revealed the true depth of my emotions to friends—even to my family. It felt as though I could count those moments when I exposed how I was truly feeling on a single hand. One was when I was diagnosed; another was when I saw my grandmother and realized how ill she was. I tried so hard to be strong for everyone, to make what was happening easy for them, even at my own expense.

But I knew I was like my grandmother. My mom told my grand-mother that as long as she wasn't able to move around independently, she wouldn't be discharged and allowed to go home. So at mealtimes when the nurses tried to coax her into a wheelchair to make the trip to the cafeteria, Grandma refused to get into it and insisted on walking down by herself. The nurses didn't like that, because it took Grandma longer, but Grandma's stubbornness paid off and eventually they discharged her. (Either that or they didn't want to deal with her anymore. I loved that about her. And I took inspiration from her.)

I wouldn't choose to go back to life before cancer. I remember reading a book by a well-known athlete who had survived the disease, and he said that he felt lucky to have been diagnosed with cancer, that he never found himself wishing it hadn't happened. I never understood that notion before—found it inconceivable—but now I do understand. Having to struggle with this disease changed me in ways that were unthinkable. I am stronger. I am resilient. I have met amazing people I wouldn't have met otherwise. And because I have seen some truly dark days, every day since then has been that much brighter.

Things have changed in other ways I could never have imagined before all of this. Greg and I moved into our new house, but we didn't live together there for long. I wanted to get out into the world and *do* things with the rest of the life I'd been granted. Greg, meanwhile, had found his spot to settle in and relax after such an ordeal. We were there in that house, but we had started to grow in different directions.

I took on some other jobs. During our first summer in our new home, I started waitressing a couple of evenings during the week and working at a winery on Sunday afternoons. Money was tight with this big new house. And Greg and I started spending less and less time together. I couldn't help but think that our relationship just wasn't what it was supposed to be. That I didn't want to spend any of the extra time I'd been granted in an unhappy marriage. Before we'd lived in our new home for even a year, it was up for sale. We divorced after a couple of years of separation. We co-parent Charley and Rudy as best we can—but we're on a new journey now, each of us going our own way.

I continued to have follow-up appointments. The first was three months after the last chemo appointment, the next was six months after, then nine months after, then just once a year. After five years, I'd be discharged, but I always joked with the doctors and nurses that I wouldn't let that happen—I felt great comfort knowing they were watching over me. Even still, I was anxious before each appointment. I was terrified they were going to tell me that the cancer had come back. But every time, they gave me the all clear.

About six months before my five-year checkup, Helen, the metformin trials nurse, called me in. She told me they were stopping the trial because they weren't seeing any benefit for women with my type of cancer. Then another blow landed. My oncology team was discharging me early. I started crying. I was scared. They were my security blanket, and I didn't know what I would do without them. They explained that what was happening was a good thing: it meant that I was okay, that I didn't have cancer anymore.

I knew that I needed to embrace that and be happy, but it was a sad day for me. I wasn't ready to let go of a piece of my life that forever changed who I am. But I hugged everyone and said my good-byes.

I am much happier now, six years down the road, although it's not all rainbows and unicorns, of course—that's just not realistic. It's hard being a single parent. It's hard not having someone to help around the house. Some of my friends have fallen by the wayside—I'm a different person than I was six years ago. I didn't choose this path, it chose me, and I became the only person that I knew how to be after going through such a traumatic life event.

I have learned that I can't make everyone happy. I am in control of nothing but my own happiness. And so that's what I try to focus on: my happiness and the happiness of my kids. I still think about my kids not having me around should cancer ever creep its way back into my life. And I immediately start to sob. Then I have to regroup and think of something else, because I simply cannot bear the thought of them alone in the world without a mother. I keep doing what I do: I keep busy. More busy than I have time for: I teach full-time, I sell real estate on the side, I write, I'm Dance Mom and Hockey Mom. And I console and embrace every new person who approaches me or gets directed my way because they just got diagnosed with cancer. I don't ever say no; I won't ever say no. I just can't, because no one ever told me they didn't have time for me when I was struggling with cancer.

I have to preach the positive because that allows me to not think about my own fate. Every time I meet someone in the same situation, though, I get jolted back to when I was diagnosed, and it's incredibly hard—I know what they're feeling and I can see the fear in their eyes. I tell them that it's all going to be okay, but I really don't know if this is true. We are all just doing the best we can.

I had this realization when I watched my friend Talia having the same experience I'd had. When I was a four-year survivor, Talia had been diagnosed with the exact same thing I'd had. She was thirty-eight years old, twenty weeks pregnant, with a nine-month-old daughter at home. I consoled her, coached her, and told her that it was going to be okay. Just one year after she was given the all clear, the cancer spread to her lungs, and there was nothing the doctors could do. Less than a year later, she passed away. Going to the funeral home was one of the most difficult moments in my life. I had told her it would all be okay. She was gone and I wasn't, and I felt guilty. Why not me? Why her?

To this day I don't know the answer, and I never will. But I do know that I have to make the best of every moment, every single opportunity, enjoy my kids every single second I can, because she can't. It's not fair, but I can't change it.

There are days when I'm having a plain old horrible day, and then I think of Talia, and I know that my horrible day isn't so bad. I am in a place in my life where I feel blessed. My mom is my rock, and always will be. I look at Charley, and while she is only ten years old, I see the beautiful, talented and fiery young woman she will become. And I look at Rudy, whose quirky ways make me laugh, and who at seven makes me stand back in awe of his natural athletic talent. I don't want to miss this. I don't want to miss *any* of this.

And so I can't help but think, often, after all I've been through and after all this time, back to when I was asked for a favor by a former student. He was playing for the local Junior B hockey team and wanted me to drop the puck at a hockey game in support of breast cancer research. It was just after all of my treatments and surgeries were done, and I was so honored. It was October. The players all wore pink, and I felt a little like a celebrity, and more important, like an advocate. I had survived and I had stories to tell that could maybe help other women.

It was an incredible experience. I drove home after the game elated and rejuvenated. Before I jumped in the shower that night, I noticed the stamp I'd gotten on my hand when I entered the arena. It was the word *Believe*. I thought about the hats I'd had made, about my determination to get through everything, to be positive, to survive. To me, that stamp wasn't just a coincidence; it was an affirmation that I was going to be okay. That everything was going to be okay.

Believe.

Acknowledgments

I am grateful for the people in my life who dropped everything to help me during my illness. I never imagined cancer would take me down the paths that it did, and in many ways I am grateful for the opportunities my illness presented me with, but I couldn't have done it without the support of everyone in my life. There are so many people who believed in the possibilities of this book before I even believed in it myself. I didn't think I had time to write a book, much less the ability, but they all helped make it happen.

Charley and Rudy: You are the reason I fought every single day. You are the reason I went to every single chemotherapy appointment even though I didn't want to endure the side effects. You are the reason I was so aggressive with my treatment schedules and so assertive with my doctors. You are the reason I decided to have a mastectomy, because I didn't want you to have to watch me ever go through that again. And you are the reason I wrote this book, because in the end, if I wasn't able to tell you this story in person, I wanted you to know without a doubt that I fought every single second of my illness for you. You are my world. You both amaze me every single day, and I don't want to miss a single minute. I love you!

Mom: You are my rock, my strength and my battery when I need recharging. You taught me how to fight like a warrior. You were there as my advocate whenever I needed you, and you were always willing to drop everything to help. You gave me the self-confidence in life to believe in the impossible and to believe that I can conquer anything. And I did. I aspire to be the amazing woman and mother that you are.

Dad: Thank you for being there for me when I was feeling my worst. You allowed me to see your fear, and I appreciated that because you were honest enough to reveal how tough this was for you. And that made me all the more determined to survive.

Erin, Doug, Jack and Natalie: Thank you for being there for me in so many ways, from the drives to and from appointments, to the leg massages when I was too achy to sleep, to the celebratory signs, balloons and cupcakes at the end of chemo. I couldn't have done any of this without that.

Braden: Even though you were far away during this time, I felt as though you were with me because of all the phone calls and e-mails from you, Erin, Isabelle, and Thomas. I know you were sending good vibes my way.

My grandmother: I miss you and think of you every day. You were the one person around whom I could let down my guard. I inherited my strength and zest for life from you. Thank you, Grandma!

Greg: It certainly has been a bumpy few years for us. Although things weren't perfect before I was diagnosed, having cancer put a strain on our relationship that we just weren't capable of handling. Thank you for trying to be there for me when I was sick; I know that being the spouse of a cancer patient was tough on you. I'm sorry you had to go through that. However, on the bright side, Charley and Rudy are who they are because of both of us, and I don't regret one bit that you are their father, because without you, they wouldn't be here, and I can't imagine life without them.

Michael and Andre: You hopped on board with the haircutting party without thinking twice. You threw one hell of a party, you had my back, and I will never forget that.

The Dinner Club: You know who you are. What a wonderful, generous, thoughtful, practical and delicious way to help someone who is going through an illness such as cancer. Kelly, you spearheaded it, and I so appreciate all of the thought and time that went into feeding me and my family. To other friends and family who dropped off meals, I cannot thank you enough.

Lepa: Thank you for cutting my hair at the party and for helping me to get it back to where it is now. You wanted me to be comfortable and to still feel like a woman. You had a profound effect on my self-esteem through the bad times, and I am so appreciative.

Kyla Gutsche: You are the most talented, meticulous and generous woman I have ever met. You made me feel confident and gave me back something I never imagined I could have. I simply cannot express what you have done for me. You changed my life.

Kim Cartmell from Focus on You Photography: Thank you for believing in the possibility of a story, and for wanting to document my journey through photos. I am so grateful for those images. Without them I wouldn't be able to reflect on those darker times; they now often seem like a distant memory, but when I look back using them, every day seems so much brighter.

Paul Tritton from Brock University Printing and Digital Services: You were so supportive of this book from the very beginning. You were always available, and I very much appreciate the time you spent on it.

Julie from Vander Brand: Thank you for your incredible attention to detail and the time and energy you put into helping me on the early incarnation of this book. Your work is unparalleled.

Talia: I think of you often. You were the bravest woman I have ever known. It's not fair what happened. The only thing that I can take from this is that I will not let a second of my life pass by unappreciated. I know you would have done the same, had you been given the opportunity.

Jeremy (Captain) Cammy: Thank you for believing in me. You didn't have to. You could have pushed me away. But you saw something—exactly what I wanted the world to see—and I am so grateful that you took that leap of faith. Or maybe I was just driving you nuts with my frequent office visits! But thank you for the conversations and the direction, and for giving me the opportunity to pitch my story to you. I am forever grateful.

Bryce, your patience and support have been paramount. You believed in the possibility of this book from the first time I pitched it to you, and you supported my quest every single second—even though I was often in need of reassurance, which you were always quick to provide. You kept me focused and positive when I needed that, and I appreciate more than you can imagine that you believed in the possibility and that you believed in me.

I would like to extend a huge thank you to Kevin Hanson and Nita Pronovost and the team at Simon & Schuster Canada. Without you, I wouldn't have been able to get this story out to as many readers as I truly believe it should get to.

To my right-hand girl, Laurie Grassi: What better editor could a writer have asked for? To say that it was a perfect fit would be the understatement of the century. Your vision for this book has been everything I could have imagined and more, and I can't thank you enough for enabling my voice to come through. You encouraged me to expand when I didn't think I had more to say, and helped me make it just right. Thank you for everything. This book wouldn't be what it is without you.

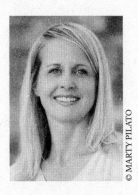

© MARTY PILATO

Born and raised in Niagara-on-the-Lake, Ontario, and still living in southwestern Ontario, Alana Somerville is a mother of two, a teacher, and a real estate sales representative. Never one to sit still, when she isn't teaching, she can often be found with her children at a hockey arena or at a dance rehearsal or on a soccer field. She also enjoys the outdoors and tries to get outside whenever possible.

Her children are her number one priority, and her drive for life is greatly inspired by them.

To find out more about Alana, visit alanasomerville.com or Twitter, @AlanaSomerville.